The Mind-Body-Spirit Connection

In The Medicine Of Light

Bernard J Fleury

Bernard J. Fleury, Ed.D.

Kurt E. Miller, Technology Consultant.

Printed by Create Space, an Amazon.com Company.

ISBN-13: 978-1729577219

ISBN-10: 1729577210

Website: www.intolifebylight.com
Printed in the United States of America

Disclaimer

I, Bernard J. Fleury, Ed.D. am not a medical doctor, so this book is not intended as medical advice of any kind such as to prevent, diagnose, treat, or cure a disease. I am educated at the graduate level in social sciences research. (See **"My Credentials"** in Part Three of this e-book).

This book is intended to share my research and experience in the medicine of light. I wrote it to share that information, for educational purposes **only,** with my readers.

This book is not intended in any way to substitute for professional medical care.

Dedication

To my Optometrist and friend
Dr. Earl Lizotte who introduced
me to Photo Dynamic Therapy

and

To David Tumey, brilliant engineer,
inventor, and friend who played a major role
in my research that led to the contents
of this e-book.

TABLE OF CONTENTS

Author:
- Meet Bernard Video at http://www.intolifebylight.com
- LinkedIn Profile at
  www.linkedin.com/pub/bernard-fleury/41/115/a44/
- Amazon Profile at
  www.amazon.com/author/bernardfleury

Please Note that a Table of Contents for each of the five E-Books/Audio Books in the Series will be on website http://www.intolifebylight.com as each E-Book/Audio Book is published.

E-Book/Audio Book One: *How Jesus Christ Leads Us to the Kingdom of Heaven.* (Published)

E-Book/Audio Book Two: How *The Mind-Body-Spirit Connection in the Medicine of Light* affects medical practice and technology that promotes my well being. (Published)

E-Book/Audio Book Three: What does *The Search for the Light in Evolution* reveal about my place as a human person in the development of the Earth?

E-Book/Audio Book Four: How does *Out of the Darkness into the Light* reflect what happens to persons who have had a profound near-death experience that really happens to *me* when I die?

E-Book/Audio Book Five: What does *The Unfailing Light* reveal that helps me deal with Alienation, Loneliness, and Depression?

In the first E-Book/Audio Book in the Called into Life by the Light Series we explored our Faith Journey with ***How Jesus Christ Leads Us To The Kingdom of Heaven.***

In this second E-Book/Audio Book in the Light Series, *The Mind-Body-Spirit Connection in the Medicine of Light*, the cover image tells us the scope of this e-book. The "head" represents the *body*, the *brain* is the *mind,* and the *Light* emanating from the inner part of the *brain* represents the *seat* of the *soul*, the spirit, the *inner light.*

Nearly every form of the outer and inner light is to be found in this e-book and audio book.

It is truly a self-help and self-understanding guide to a healthier life.

Reviews

The Mind-Body-Spirit in the Medicine of Light by Bernard Fleury is the second book in the Called into Life by the Light Series. The author seeks to educate and inform the reader of the history and benefits of light therapy, whether it is being used to combat seasonal depression or to soothe agitated behavior. It is written in an easy to understand way so that anyone from a health care professional to a layperson can readily understand the information that Bernard offers, which is full of convincing evidence as to the benefits of light medicine. But, overall, Fleury encourages self agency and self advocacy in the hope that the reader opens their mind to new alternatives to healing.

I found The Mind-Body-Spirit in the Medicine of Light by Bernard Fleury to be well written and informative. It is written in a way that makes for easy consumption and understanding, while at the same time provides gems for all aspects of life. Fleury offers a convincing array of evidence from several sources, and the knowledge provides many tools that the reader can use to grow and thrive. And while Fleury has crafted such an engaging book, it's also a dense read. Luckily, it's broken down into easy to digest parts that will, nonetheless, stick with the reader for a long time, providing content that is guaranteed to be reread and pored over. The final few pages are filled with recommendations to other works that have helped the author and, hopefully, the reader. Great for anyone looking for a change in their life.

Reviewer: Kayti Nika Raet, Readers' Favorite, Rating *****

The Mind-Body-Spirit in the Medicine of Light is the second book in the Called into Life by the Light Series by Bernard Fleury, a book with a content that is aptly captured in its title. In this book, the author explores the connection between mind, body, and soul and how mastering this connection can ensure inner peace, harmony, robust health, and fullness of life. Having experienced the phenomenon of light in its diverse forms, the author began a journey which would lead him to uncover the treasures in light and its healing energy. In this book, the author explores a new way of diagnosis and treatment for a variety of illnesses, sharing with readers powerful medical concepts related to light, the place of the eyes as the windows of the soul, and a lot more.

This book discusses modern medical procedures that use light and advanced devices to diagnose and treat different kinds of illnesses. The methods used in the modern treatments are less invasive, more accurate in diagnosis, and most effective when it comes to actual treatment, which has no life-threatening effects. This is one of the first medical books I have read that offers methods combining science and a holistic approach to treatment in a stunning manner. There is a spiritual as well as a philosophical aspect of this book that readers will enjoy as well. The book is well-researched and offers surprising discoveries about the energy of light, which comes primarily from the sun and is present in different life forms. This isn't just a book for people seeking to be cured of an illness, but one that proposes a path to general wellness and wholeness of mind, body, and spirit. The Mind-Body-Spirit in the Medicine of Light is informative, a book that explores the mystery of life from a fresh and unique perspective. Bernard Fleury's book is a gift for those who want to experience life deeply.

Reviewer: Ruffina Oserio, Readers' Favorite, Rating *****

There is more to light than just what we may think, and in The Mind-Body-Spirit in the Medicine of Light by Bernard J. Fleury you will discover much of what light is really about. It's a way of helping you to see more deeply into your own body and even those around you. But it's also a way of healing and empowering yourself. When we allow our eyes to use that light and to simply show us what we need to know, we can harness these abilities fully. Researchers throughout history have sought to understand light. They've sought to understand how it impacts the body and the mind, and what they have found is remarkable. Light is a way for the body to accomplish much more than we had previously thought.

This book is all about the power of light and the way that it can help the body to heal and to become stronger. Light has been used as a method of treatment and medicine since ancient history, though people then may not have truly understood what they were doing at the time. In this book you find out more about how light has been used and continues to be used. As we come to recognize even more capabilities from light, scientists are starting to develop additional treatments and ways to harness its abilities with light therapy. Once we do, it's possible to truly achieve the best for ourselves. There's definitely more to be discovered, but The Mind-Body-Spirit in the Medicine of Light is a great start.

Reviewer: Samantha Dewitt (Rivera), Readers' Favorite Rating *****

Description

Light based medicine is painless and heals without side effects that are worse than the disease being treated. **What if** you can get accurate diagnosis of many diseases with an MRI, CT scanner or Ultra-sound usually with minimal or no side effects? **What if** you can improve your eyesight with phototherapy with no side effects? **What if** you discover that there was a cancer cure that worked since its discovery in the summer of 1934 at the first cancer clinic using Royal Raymond Rife's technology? **What if** you discover why this treatment is available in Germany but is restricted to animals in the United States?

The Mind-Body-Spirit Connection in the *Medicine of Light* is the second e-Book and Audio Book in the Called into Life by the Light Series of five e-Books and Audio Books.

Part One is a detailed expansion of Chapter IV: *The Medicine of Light* from the 2009 print book *Called into Life by the Light*, which was suppressed in April 2013.

Part Two is the script of the one hour conversation I had with David Tumey on June 6, 2012. We discussed David's part in rediscovering Royal R. Rife's Ray Tube, reconstructing Rife's 1950's instrument, and shortening the time factor in producing the correct frequency, MOR (Mortal Oscillatory Rate) which would devitalize (destroy) a particular cancer. The reader/listener will also read or hear of David's continuing efforts in this area as of July 21, 2013 when he updated parts of the June 6, 2012 conversation.

Part Three is about Royal R. Rife, The timeline of his life, his Beam Ray Instrument, Universal Microscope, and BX, The Cancer Causing Microbe.

Part Four is an update on Royal R. Rife's Technology and Influence in 2014.

Purpose Statement

I have created this e-book because I want to inform others of the revolution that we are experiencing in the Medicine of Light in terms of therapies like Photo Dynamic Therapy and devices like the Magnetic Resonance Imaging (MRI) scanner which creates an image of the area being scanned and displays it on a computer monitor.

Photo Dynamic Therapies and the devices used to implement them are all light based. They work because they reflect the basic stuff of the universe in one or another if its forms of light like magnetic fields and radio waves.

These therapies and devices are the least invasive and most effective of modern medical ways of diagnosis and treatment. They are also the most effective in terms of accurate diagnosis which leads to the best available, least invasive, and most effective treatment with no life threatening side effects. In short, the side effects of the prescribed treatment are not more lethal than those of the disease being treated!

Preface

The first e-book and audio book in the Called into Life Series is *How Jesus Christ Leads Us to the Kingdom of Heaven.* We read or heard and pondered the many inspirational Bible verses in both the Old and New Testaments on life and light. We discovered how life and light in the Bible are really tied together (lifelight), with The Light, Jesus Christ, being the guide and sustainer in life's journey of Spiritual Growth in Christian Living. Union with The Light in the heavenly Jerusalem, the Kingdom of Heaven is the ultimate fulfillment, the goal of every human life.

In this second e-book and audio book in the Light Series, *The Mind-Body-Spirit Connection in the Medicine of Light*, the cover image tells us the scope of this e-book. The "head" represents the *body*, the *brain* is the *mind*, and the *Light* emanating from the inner part of the *brain* represents the *seat* of the *soul*, the *spirit*, the *inner light.*

Nearly every form of the outer and inner light is to be found in this e-book and audio book.

It is truly a self-help and self-understanding guide to a healthier life.

PART ONE: THE MEDICINE OF LIGHT

Long before I was involved in a serious study of the phenomenon of light, I recognized in myself an intense sensitivity to light in all its forms. From my recollection of the early years of my life, my sleep patterns have always been highly affected by light. If I had been sleeping for eight hours or so before the time of my rising, and the rising time was prior to natural daylight, I found it very difficult to get out of bed and that is still the case. As I am aging into my early eighties my body clock winds down sooner at the end of natural daylight but awakens as soon as natural daylight. But the clock comes streaming into my bedroom window.

I have always wanted to be in natural daylight as much as possible during the day outdoors. If indoors, I liked working by a window with abundant natural light. My career as a public school teacher and college professor found me maximizing natural light in my classrooms and requesting office space with abundant windows as sources of natural light. I seldom turned on the artificial lights, which were either incandescent or limited-spectrum fluorescent. I was forced to do so by natural darkness when my work schedule kept me there past the end of daylight. I have always felt good in the light. It has been a lifelong medicine for me.

In 1993, due to a persistent "lazy eye" condition in my right eye and the beginning deterioration in acuity of vision in my left eye, I sought a new phototherapy treatment recommended by my Optometrist, Dr. Earl Lizotte, who had been working in the field of Syntonic Optometry since the late 1980's. It was during this treatment that I was told of the work of Dr. Jacob Liberman and made aware of his book, *Light Medicine of the Future.* Dr. Lizotte was also exploring the work of Arthur Zajonc on the history of light as described in Zajonc's 1993 book, *Catching the Light.* `In the Forward to Jacob Liberman's book, *Light - Medicine of the Future,* John Ott, a pioneer in the field of photobiology, asks the question

14

"Are we to totally discount our own abilities to see, hear, and feel our everyday experience, trusting only the findings of others who differ from us in their view of reality?" (Jacob Lieberman, *Light Medicine of the Future* page xv). The "real" is often hidden beneath the exceptional. The optical illusions researched by Goethe were accurate illustrations of the behavior of light. We must be open to new insights. Present day scientific methods are not eternal. They do not have the final answer and so cannot be allowed to be an *absolute* norm for what is scientific.

Dr. Jacob Liberman is a pioneer in the fields of light, vision and consciousness, and author of *Light Medicine of the Future, Take Off Your Glasses and See,* and *Wisdom From an Empty Mind.* He earned a Doctorate of Optometry from Southern College of Optometry, a Ph.D. in Vision Science from the College of Syntonic Optometry, and was awarded an Honorary Doctorate of Science from the Open International University for Complementary Medicines. He is a Fellow Emeritus of the American Academy of Optometry, College of Optometrists in Vision Development, College of Syntonic Optometry and International Academy of Color Sciences, and Past President of the College of Syntonic Optometry. He is also the recipient of the H.R. Spitler Award for his pioneering contributions to the field of Phototherapy. Dr. Liberman has shared his discoveries and insights with more than 2,000 audiences worldwide and been enthusiastically endorsed by luminaries in the fields of health, science, spirituality and sports. He is the inventor of the Color Receptivity Trainer, Spectral Receptivity System and *EYEPORT Vision Training System,* the first FDA-cleared medical device that significantly improves visual performance. Dr. Liberman is the Founder of *Exercise Your Eyes, Inc.* and President of the *International Society For The Study Of Subtle Energies And Energy Medicine* (ISSSEEM). He is a faculty member of the *Institute for Scientific Exploration* and serves on the advisory board of the *Institute for Science, Spirituality and Sustainability.* His most recent project, EYELIGHT, will revolutionize our understanding of how light interacts with the body evaluating the composition of light entering and exiting the eyes. He was also president of Universal Light Technologies Limited, a company that researched and developed photo therapeutic devices for healing.

His approach integrates scientific research, clinical experience, and his own intuitive insights. The college that he led has advocated the use of light therapy by way of the eyes since its inception in the 1930's. (255) His own painful life experiences led him to a number of insights. First of all, he states that most of what life reveals to us comes when we are not looking for anything specific. In fact when we are too specific, too narrow in terms of what we are looking for, we tend to miss everything we were not looking for. "People are meant to see passively not actively,...our eyes are meant to see for us, if we let them...vision is meant to be effortless" (xx). As a result of this insight he stopped wearing glasses and began to actively experiment with the workings of his mind, especially with the integration of mind and eyes, the relationship between the inner and the outer light.

...“if we allow our eyes to see for us as they are meant to see, they will always bring our attention to anything in the environment that is out of place or not flowing with that experience" (xx). We need to step back like the artist does who is in the midst of a painting, to look at the whole work, not anything in particular—to just let our eyes do what they are supposed to do, see for us. Liberman began to utilize this insight in his clinical practice by just casually gazing at his patients during initial treatment sessions, allowing his eyes to fall where they might on various parts of patient's bodies. He felt that "something seemed to be stuck there and that the body's energy appeared to be rerouted through an adjacent area" (xxi). Upon questioning these patients he found that their problems were located in the body parts upon which his eyes had fallen intuitively.

In 1977 he learned of a specific form of light therapy called Syntonics that "therapeutically utilizes different portions of the visible light spectrum to treat, by way of the

16

eyes, an array of bodily conditions" (xxi). He attended a course at the College of Syntonic Optometry and thus began his life's work. Liberman concludes the Preface to his book with a concise statement of the basic assumptions upon which his book is written: "Our task is to take in and utilize light so that we may merge with our true selves and our destiny, thus facilitating the healing of our planet. As each of us becomes whole, we radiate light—light from within—unimpeded by our self- imposed emotional and physical blocks. The medicine of the future is light. We are healing ourselves with that which is our essence" (xxii).

His book is all about the science of light, a science that synthesizes scientific knowledge, intuitive knowing, health, and personal evolution. Liberman uses the term "science" in its original Latin derivation, that is, "knowledge" and he includes induction, deduction, and intuition as all equal and reliable ways of knowing. He appears to rely most heavily on intuition as the beginning of the scientific process. That is not an unusual stance. In the late nineteenth century, the great philosopher and educator, John Dewey, wrote that all knowing, all science, begins with a hunch, a felt need, an intuition. Further thought and refinement of that hunch results in one or more hypotheses which are then experimentally affirmed or rejected by means of the remaining steps of the scientific method. Liberman maintains that the synthesized nature of the science of light provides a new paradigm in healing. He writes that light is at the core of the new "energy medicine" of the 1990's.

…"light is the basic component from which all life originates, develops, heals, evolves…we are about to see a new marriage between the 'intuitive' and the 'rational' sciences—a marriage that is *bonded* by light…Miracle after miracle has convinced me that this science of the future is an investigation of inner space rather than outer space" (xxv).

Dan Millman, world champion gymnast, explorer of various wisdom traditions, noted author of 17 books in the

Peaceful Warrior Series, and quoted in Liberman's biographical article cited in Wikipedia, writes, "Dr. Jacob Liberman is at the cutting edge of enlightened technology blending physics and metaphysics to their best advantage." In other words, Liberman is a great synthesizer. He looks at things from various perspectives like the two he lists about Liberman's physics and metaphysics.

Liberman presents *Light - Medicine of the Future* in fifteen chapters, the titles of which I will utilize in organizing my summarization and analysis of his work.

The Human Photocell

That the human body is a living photocell, energized and controlled by light entering the eyes, is one of Liberman's basic and innovative assumptions. (xxv) Once this light enters the body it has a profound effect on both our physiological and emotional functioning as well as the development of our awareness. Our lives are truly dependent on the sun and the small portion of its electromagnetic waves that reach our planet. The approximately one percent of these waves which reach us and are visible, are essential to proper human functioning and evolution.

Liberman repeats physicist David Bohm's postulate that "all matter is frozen light." Light is all in all, the basic stuff of the universe that manifests itself in a variety of forms. He joins Teilhard de Chardin and Arthur Zajonc in asking whether the evolution of humans both individually and collectively, has basically been dependent on our ability to receive and to make use of both the inner and outer lights, the "within" and the "without," the spiritual and the physical. As both Teilhard and Arthur Zajonc have stated, the inner light is crucial because it gives meaning to what we physically see.

The rhythm of life is directly affected by light in the sequence of night, day, and the seasons. Sunrise marks a period

18

of transition and new beginnings—from rest to activity. Yellow (sun), blue (sky), green (earth), mark the day. Red orange (sunset) changing into dark blue (night) marks the transition from day to night. At the exact point of sunset, a flash of green is often seen—green, the center of the visible spectrum, the flash that indicates a passing of one phase prior to entering a new phase of functioning/living. I have personally observed this flash of green several times over the years as the sun goes down over the Caribbean Sea in Grand Cayman. It is a brilliant but instantaneous transition from day to night.

Seasonal color changes reflect and affect biological alterations in all living things. The soft greens and the other pastels of spring affect plant growth, flowering, and the breeding habits of all living things including humans. Summer brings with it more intense colors, darker green, more yellows and oranges in flowers, the time for birth for many reptiles and mammals and for growing and maturing. Autumn finds the landscape (in temperate zones at least) flooded with warm colors of red, yellow, orange, as well as the earthy tones of various shades of brown as nature prepares for rest. The cool whites, blues, etc., of winter indicate a restfulness, a time to regroup. But the decreased exposure to sunlight especially in areas near the poles results in a dramatic increase in irritability, fatigue, illness, insomnia, depression, alcoholism, and suicide, as Liberman asserts, and statistics verify. (7)

From ancient times, the Sun has been recognized as the original healer. The Egyptians, Romans, and Greeks, among others made medical use of light. Color, a manifestation of light, held a therapeutic as well as divine meaning for these cultures as you can read in Zajonc's work, *Catching the Light*. Beginning as early as 1796 in the work of Hufeland, modern science began to recognize the value of light in medicine. Hufeland noted the effects of the deprivation of light on prisoners kept in the dark—their bodies grow pale and soft, their minds apathetic, gradually losing all their vital energy. These same phenomena are being observed in persons who spend most of their lives indoors under limited spectrum florescent lights.

In *Introduction to a Submolecular Biology, and Bioelectronics,* Albert Szent-Gyorgyi, Nobel Prize winner and discoverer of vitamin C came to the following conclusions:

1. All the energy we take into our bodies is derived from the sun.
2. The sun's energy, stored in plants, eaten by animals and humans, digested by breaking down and utilizing this light-created energy.
3. Many enzymes and hormones involved in processing this energy are colored and very sensitive to light.
4. Light striking the body can literally alter the basic biological functions involved in processing the body's fuel, which powers our lives. [23]

The dramatic effect of light on bodily functioning was borne out by the conclusions of others as well, including the work of Martinek and Berezin in 1979 and Dr. Zane Kime. Martinek and Berezin reported in the March 1979 issue of *Photochemistry and Photobiology* that:

1. Some colors of light can stimulate enzymes to be five-hundred percent more effective;
2. Some colors can increase the rate of enzymatic reactions, activate or deactivate certain enzymes, and affect the movement of substances across cell membranes. [4]

Dr. Zane Kime's experiments as reported in his book, *Sunlight,* seem to indicate that the human body behaves like a living photocell. It is energized by the sun's light. After a planned pattern of exposure to sunlight, the body reacted in specific ways following exercise. Decreases were noted in resting heart rate, blood pressure, etc., and increases in energy, strength and ability of blood to absorb and carry oxygen. [5]

The Eyes Are the Windows of the Soul

Our eyes provide the means for the interrelationship of the world without and the world within. We meet persons and objects and show how we feel with our eyes. Liberman begins this chapter with the statement that our eyes reflect our physical and emotional health by serving as an index of many different physical health functions or conditions, and are accurate indicators of mental states and styles of operation.

The eyes serve as the major gateways through which light enters and affects the body's total functioning including consciousness. The Gospel of Luke relates: "The light of the body is your eye, when your eye is clear, your whole body is clear, your whole body is also full of light; but when it is bad, your body is full of darkness" (Luke 11:34). The present-day clinical science of iridology, which many still consider a pseudoscience, is based on the assumption that the iris of the eye is a real map of the body; that each section of the iris correlates with a specific part/organ of the body. Liberman cites the findings of a group of Russian scientists, reported in 1989, which found a one-hundred-percent correlation between the diagnosis of their iridodiagnostic technique and the actual physical conditions of their subjects. [6]

It is very interesting to note that the principal conveyors of light to us are really extensions of our brains, the most complex (most parts) of any currently known human system. Brain and eye weight is two percent of our total weight but they require a quarter of our nutritional energy, a major part of our oxygen, vitamin C, and zinc intakes. Our eyes contain seventy percent of the body's sense receptors, and except in the case of totally blind persons, provide access for approximately ninety percent of all we learn in our lifetime. (16)

As we have already noted, modern science is looking at the eyes as the "gateways of the mind." Liberman believes that specific mental patterns are directly related to the functioning or dysfunctioning of the physical eye, and light has a direct effect on our mental states. (18) Light is *the* principal nurturer of our bodies having a vital effect on our physical and emotional functions. Although hypothesized and tested since the late 1800's, it wasn't until the early 1970's that it was finally proven definitively, that when light entered the eyes, it didn't only affect seeing, but also affected the brain's hypothalamus, which in turn is the coordinator and regulator of most of our life-support functions. It also initiates and directs our reactions and adaptations to stress. (22-25) The Greeks and other ancient civilizations knew this and practiced it in their medicine. Now we have scientifically confirmed that the nervous and endocrine systems are directly stimulated and regulated by light to an extent not accepted, until recently by modern science. (22)

The Pineal: Seat of the Soul

The Pineal, which in humans, is a small pea sized gland located deep in the center of the brain between the two hemispheres and behind and above the pituitary gland, was considered in the early Twentieth Century to be vestigial like our tonsils, with no real purpose. It is now believed that the pineal is the body's master regulator, receiving light activated information from the eyes by way of the hypothalamus. It then transmits this information to the rest of the body telling whether it is daylight or darkness, and how long the days are. Animals that are more directly in touch with their environment (sunlight and the outdoors) than most modern humans, tend to have larger pineal glands. Liberman asks whether a change in our consciousness, and a closer connection between us and nature would increase the size of our pineal? (31)

In birds, lizards, and fish, the skull serves as a third eye through which light enters the body, but this is not presently true for humans. Light enters our bodies by way of our eyes—it affects our eyes and our hypothalamus gland that in turn affects the Pineal. The Pineal releases a very powerful hormone, melatonin, that can be found everywhere in the body and affects all bodily functions. Melatonin is secreted in response to darkness, and if we are exposed to light for an hour or more its levels change in response to two hundred to six hundred lux of light. A lux equals approximately the light of one candle. Liberman writes that every cell in the body is influenced by light striking the eyes. Because of our bodies reaction to light our biological rhythms run smoothly. (32)

Dr. Fritz Hollwich, (researcher, author, former professor of ophthalmology at the University of Muenster in Germany) confirmed in 1979, that stimulatory and regulatory effects of light on the human body take place by way of the eyes— absent light perception and physiological and emotional stability is greatly reduced. The Pineal is the regulator of regulators. It affects reproduction, growth, body temperature, blood pressure, motor activity, sleep, tumor growth, mood, the immune system, and even longevity! (33)

Liberman concludes this chapter by stating that the hypothalamus is the interfacer and coordinator between mind and body, affecting our vital functions, consciousness, and preparedness, with the environmental conditions to which we are exposed. We become part of this environment. (36)

But how do we synchronize our bodies with the environment so that we become one with the process of evolution going on in the universe? We are really asking how can we integrate the inner and outer person, the light within and the light without, the mind (head and reason) with the body (solar plexus and intuition-felt sense), the spirit and the flesh, science and religion?

In their book, *Bio-Spirituality*, Peter Campbell and Edwin McMahon, priest-therapists, workshop and retreat leaders, suggest that a process called "Focusing," as taught by Dr. Eugene

Gendlin of the University of Chicago, is a practical method of body consciousness, a searching for bodily

23

awareness, that is in fact a spiritual way of knowing—not with our minds alone, but with our bodies. Focusing is a simple way of attending to meaning that is felt in the body, the interconnectedness of mind (head, reason) and body (solar plexus-felt sense). Campbell and McMahon assert that there is "a *felt* truth, a *felt* meaning, a *felt* direction within each of us that can free us and guide us into the future. In-touch living connects! It allows values and behavior to change." [7] It allows the light within to connect with the light without.

In Appendix ii of *Bio-Spirituality,* "The interface between science and religion," the authors insist that we have to learn to see things in new ways. As in Alfred Tennyson' s poem, *The Passing of Arthur*, the dying King says: "The old order changeth, yielding place to new, and God fulfills himself in many ways"(134). Campbell and McMahon ask, "What precisely, establishes *an old order*? Is it not the way things are seen?...Are faith *and* vision somehow nurtured within the crucible of change itself? Is *believing* actually an awareness and living out of this changing perspective" (134)?

They then go on to write that there are several ways to explore this possibility, one of which is to be found in modern physics. They cite the work of the critical realist physicist, David Bohm, that light resists the attempt to be split into "atomic pieces." The most fundamental feature of light is its wholeness. It can be one and many, particle and wave, a single thing but with a universe inside.

The photographic process called Holography which produces a three dimensional image called a hologram was part of Bohm's investigations. The fascinating aspect of the hologram is that it stores information in a way totally unlike conventional photography.

If a small piece is broken or cut from the holographic plate and the same wave-length of laser light is directed toward this divided portion, *the entire original scene can still be seen through this smaller segment of the transparency.* This happens because information about the total scene is present within every part of the hologram. *The whole is contained in each part of the holographic image...*All of the whole is within every part. [8]

Experiments like Bohm's challenge our every day perceptions of reality especially the lack of unity these perceptions present initially to our senses. Bohm suggests that we view the structure of the universe as holographic with its entire *explicate* structure (the "without," that is, particles, multiplicity), encoded in its every part. Each natural unit is a microcosm of the whole universe. Since this is so, Bohm posits a further order, an *implicate* order, the order of undivided wholeness. One does not have to believe in a world of one *or* a world of many. Both beliefs are valid and interact with each other in an orderly constructive fashion. (138)

> Bohm then goes on to consider the actual unfolding itself, that inner *movement* from implicate to explicate which grounds an appearance of "the whole" within each part. This fundamental *movement*, we feel, is what surfaces in the Focusing process. The human organism knows its connectedness. That connectedness appears with and *as* the unfolding of each felt sense. The body's knowing of holographic tied-in-ness is expressed within the forward *movement* of felt meaning. Focusing allows this embodied sense for deeper unification to surface within the very process that carries it forward. (138)

Bohm is not content with a vague expression of an underlying unity in the universe. He has moved on to a consideration of the actual process that grounds *both* implicate and explicate orders. In an interview done by John Welwood in 1980 and published in the *Journal of Transpersonal Psychology*, Bohm names this basic energy and its movement.

"The energy which moves between the explicate and implicate orders is still further inward. It is the force that brings about the unfolding of the implicate. You see, we have the explicate order and the implicate order, and the movement from one to the other—which is *the holomovement*" (139).

The holomovement is more inward than the explicate or implicate orders; it is the ground of both. Beyond the orders and this movement, Bohm says, lies an emptiness and fullness that cannot be uttered. Campbell and McMahon ask:

Is this a physicist's way of approaching the mystic experience of God?…Is believing actually the maturing awareness which each person has of this unutterable ground of being, the holomovement and whatever lies beyond?…We ask whether there might be a special kind of consciousness that can perceive this movement, and we are suggesting that such a perspective and perception is what has been traditionally meant by believing. (140)

Reason (cognitive domain—induction, deduction) which utilizes calculation and logic, and which aims at prediction and control, is the basic stuff of scientific method. Faith involves intellectual assent but also intuition, awareness, willingness to receive, the affective domain. It looks at the remote as well as the immediate, beyond the individual life to life itself. Faith calls for an attitude of allowing, not control. It operates as Liberman says the eyes should, that is, be allowed to see what they see, and not be always limited to a specific narrow focus. Thus, believing differs essentially from reasoning not only because of its usual content (faith) but because the *way* one thinks (perceives) when *believing* is radically different from the way one thinks (perceives) when *reasoning.*

David Bohm and Teilhard de Chardin are alike in their belief that there is a precise energy at work in consciousness evolution, a process which grounds the explicate and implicate orders before fading off beyond all present knowing into some unutterable fullness...Focusing is a very practical way of allowing ourselves to be drawn forward one step at a time on the long journey into this holomovement. It is a doorway beyond reason into faith. Not faith in the sense of specific doctrines of belief, but a believing that is the gift and expression of some deeper awareness. It is letting go into the very flow of evolution that brings us home to a Greater Self-Process. (141)

Focusing can be the vehicle that helps us synchronize our inner and outer selves with our environment, the light within and the light without. We enter the holomovement that begins in light, is moved forward by light, and culminates in light.

Color: The Rainbow of Life

The opening paragraph of this chapter in Liberman's book is a powerful one that links light and life. He states that light brings to life the objects it touches and then these objects first appear as colors which become forms—our initial visual perceptions and discriminations are of color, then of form. Color has a power and language of its own. It causes us to feel excited, depressed, or peaceful. Used in advertising it can lead us to purchasing things. We speak of red hot, cool as a cucumber (green), white as a ghost, feeling blue, etc. Light is responsible for the emergence of all life, and all life literally is light.

The range of visible light for humans has been determined for us by our evolutionary development under a sun whose light reaches earth in wave lengths of 400-700NM (Nano-meters = one billionth of a meter) which are the wavelengths of visible light for us. Thus the sun has shaped our nervous systems so that we see colors only within those wave lengths.

The seasons of the year, especially in the temperate zones, illustrate the way colors are related to the growth and

27

development of all living things. Spring is the greening time—
the time for rebirth of plants and new birth of mammals—the
time for new beginnings. Summer green becomes more intense,
and the pastels of spring give way to the more vibrant colors
of summer—a time for growing. Colors become brilliant and
earthen in the fall and change rapidly, moving to the more
somber tones as winter approaches. Fall is a time for
maturing and seeing things with an evolutionary (broad
stroke—long term) perspective. Winter's colors are stark:
white, black, dark blue—cold—reflecting the death of one
phase of the year and of our lives, but also a time for resting
and introspection before the growth cycle begins again.

Liberman cites the work of Johann Wolfgang von Goethe
and Rudolph Steiner as major contributors to our
knowledge of the relationship between color, feelings and
responses, as does Arthur Zajonc in *Catching The Light*. From
1840 until the 1920's J. W. von Goethe's work on color theory,
Farbenlehre was considered the definitive work on color theory.
In 1921 Rudolph Steiner, a Goethe scholar, stated clearly in his
book *Colour,* that seen color provokes feelings that lead to our
actions. Life manifests itself in various colors, so all color is
really light, and light is both the source of life and life itself. [9]

Color preference as investigated by Dr. Max Lusher has a
definite correlation with either a state of mind or glandular
imbalance or both. We react to specific colors the way we
do because of our deeply embedded primal memory. Certain
parts of our brains are not only light sensitive but also
respond differently to different wave lengths. In the late
twentieth century, and increasingly in the twenty first
century, we are now coming to a conclusion that what
ancient Sanskrit writings describe, is true, namely, that
"different colors (wave lengths) of radiation interact
differently with the endocrine system to stimulate or inhibit
hormonal production"(43). This process may be described as
the psychophysiological effects of colors.

Beginning in 1942 a number of scientists have investigated

this process as the time line that follows indicates.

1942-1951   S. V. Krakov found that red stimulated the sympathetic portion of the autonomic nervous system and blue stimulated the parasympathetic portion.

1958   Krakov's findings confirmed by Robert Gerard: the autonomic nervous system and visual cortex were significantly less aroused when stimulated by blue or white light than when stimulated by red light.

1958   Dr. Harry Wohlfarth also used the autonomic nervous system to demonstrate that certain colors have measurable and predictable effects on humans.

1968   Dr. Jerold Lucey found that when he exposed jaundiced babies to either full spectrum light or blue light for several days, their bilirubin was lowered to safe levels. This has now become the most common form of treatment for what had been a life threatening condition. Some medical researchers now feel that jaundice in babies may be caused by the lack of sunlight in many modern windowless nurseries. Liberman thinks that the fact that more than ninety percent of our population works indoors and lacks sufficient exposure to natural light may be a significant factor in their offsprings' health.

1971   B. S. Aaronson found that specific colors affect mood, breathing rate, pulse rate, and blood pressure.

1974   B. S. Aaronson's work confirmed by J. J. Plack and J. Schick.

29

1979-1985	Schaus, Pellegrini, T. J. Birk, Gruson, and Costigan did a series of studies on the effects of the color pink on aggressive behavior in prison inmates-had a definite calming effect-small pink holding cells now used to significantly reduce the incidence of violent and aggressive behavior.
1982	Dr. Sharon McDonald, conducted an experiment on sixty middle-aged women with rheumatoid arthritis. She exposed their hands to blue light and found that this light was very effective in reducing pain-the longer the exposure, the greater the likelihood of reduced pain.
1985	Dr. John Ott filmed the effects of color on a living organism (chloroplasts) in different ways, causing them to move in different patterns or to rest. Ott demonstrated that altering plant cellular function by altering the light source affects the normal process of photosynthesis and the resulting cell chemistry.
1988	G. Legwold showed that viewing red light may assist athletic performance requiring quick bursts of energy, while blue light may assist performances requiring a more steady level of energy output.
1990	Dr. John Anderson monitored seven migraine sufferers for up to two years to evaluate the effects of blinking red lights on the severity of their migraines. Seventy-two percent of the seven reported that migraines stopped within an hour of beginning the treatment. Of the other twenty-eight percent, ninety-three percent reported feeling better.

Liberman concludes this chapter by asserting that the

type of lighting under which we live and work can, over time, cause some of the differences in behavior and physiology among humans. [10]

Malillumination: Fact or Fantasy

If light is the source of life as well as the major nutrient sustaining life, then poor or incomplete lighting must have an adverse affect on human life. Prior to the 1879 perfection of the incandescent bulb by Edison, most persons spent most of their time outdoors as most occupations and household chores like cutting wood, gardening, tending to animals, required an outdoor presence. Since that date increasing numbers of persons leaning on the illumination of the light bulb have spent ever-greater portions of each day indoors in a limited spectrum light environment.

Three kinds of artificial illumination are common today:

1. the incandescent bulb—the most commonly used source in homes—fairly complete
range of the visible color spectrum but deficient in blue end—virtually no ultraviolet light— emits much of light as yellow and red and maximum energy as infrared (heat).

2. florescent—cool white is commonest form—deficient in red and blue-violet where sun's rays are strongest.

3. high intensity discharge – used commonly as street lamps and security lights – very bright orange red or blue lights.

In a longitudinal study done by Dr. D. B. Harmon, as reported in "The Coordinated Classroom" in 1951, the effects of lighting (and other factors) on the human functioning and development of school aged children was investigated. The study began in 1938 under the auspices of the Texas Department of Health. In the first three years over one hundred sixty thousand school children were screened for health and educational problems which revealed that by the

31

completion of elementary school, over half of children had "developed an average of two observable, but preventable, deficiencies" (56). When these deficiencies were correlated with classroom factors it became evident that these "were related to bodily activities aroused when the eyes were stimulated by light" (56).

In 1942 the study focused on developing methods for controlling these adverse factors. In 1946 Harmon combined the findings and used them as the basis for recommending optimum lighting, seating, and décor, to maximize school performance with minimal effort. One of the study's schools was redone to meet these criteria, and a six- month study to test the results was undertaken. Visual difficulties, chronic fatigue, nutritional problems, and chronic infections were reduced by forty-three to sixty-five percent. (56)

Harmon's study paid more attention to light distribution rather than to the quality of light distributed. Dr. John Ott, on the other hand, concentrated his work on the relationship between the quality (type) of light and the well being of all living organisms. A banker by profession he developed his life-long interest in photography to a full-time investigation of the ecology of light. His studies were carefully designed and controlled and undertaken at several top medical schools and research hospitals.

The lifespan of experimental animals was dramatically affected by the type of lighting in their environment. Mice under pink fluorescents lived an average of 7.5 months, under daylight- white fluorescents, 8.2 months, and under natural daylight for 16.1 months—a lifespan more than double those that lived exclusively under pink or white florescent lights. Based on these results, Ott concluded that natural light was as important to the well-being of animals as it was to plants. As a result of his work and encouraged by him, Duro-Test developed the first full-spectrum florescent tube, the Vita-Lite. [11]

Ott next carried his investigations on light and life to humans. In a Florida school based experiment, two windowless classrooms were illuminated with cool white florescent lights, and two with full spectrum radiation-shielded florescent lights. In the cool white classrooms some children "demonstrated hyperactivity, fatigue, irritability, and attentional deficits"(58). In the full spectrum classrooms, behavior, classroom performance, and a reduction in hyperactivity among several learning disabled children, resulting in the resolution of some of their learning and reading problems, was noted within one month. Another interesting result was that in the full spectrum rooms children developed one-third less cavities in their teeth than did the cool white rooms children. Research conducted much earlier in the 1930's had shown that summertime with its maximum exposure to natural light saw a marked decrease in the incidence of cavities compared to the short day months. "The more sunlight, the less cavities." [12, 13]

Not only does sunlight appear to affect the incidence of cavities but in the December 8, 1987 edition of the *Wall Street Journal*, L. Hays reported that chickens raised under full spectrum lighting "live twice as long, lay more eggs, are less aggressive, and produce eggs that are approximately twenty-five percent lower in cholesterol." [14] Direct moderate exposure to sunlight both outdoors and indoors (full-spectrum light) has been shown by Altschul and Herman (1953) to significantly and rapidly reduce cholesterol levels in human beings. [15]

In a 1980 study, done by F. Hollwich and B. Dieckhues, exposure to natural versus artificial light via the eye, was shown to have dramatically different effects on the hormonal and metabolic balance of both animals and humans. One group of persons sat under cool white and the other under full spectrum artificial lighting. Stress-like levels of ACTH and cortisol (the stress hormones) were found in the cool white group and were totally absent in the full spectrum group. These findings clarify the earlier findings of Ott regarding the effects of cool white lights on the stress, fatigue, and mental capabilities of children. Liberman records that as a result of this and other research "the cool-white fluorescent bulb is legally banned in German hospitals and medical facilities." [16]

Liberman concludes this chapter with a section on using light to revitalize food and water by exposing our food during preparation time to natural sunlight or specially designed "Kiva" lights.

The Enlightened Pioneers

Light's therapeutic applications and its affect on the function of all living things have been described by a number of persons since the days of Herodotus, the father of heliotherapy. There also have been a number of persons who have investigated the scientific properties of light.

In the 1800's physicians became fully aware of the healing properties of sunlight especially with regard to tuberculosis. In the 1870's practitioners of heliotherapy began looking at color and not just direct sunlight for treatment. General Augustus Pleasanton in 1876, in his book *Blue and Sun-Lights* claimed that greenhouses paned with alternating blue and transparent glass panels increased the size, quality, and yield of grapes grown therein. He also claimed that blue light had curative effects on both animals and humans. In his book *Blue and Red Lights*, Dr. S. Pancoast in 1877, claimed that the use of sunlight filtered through panes of red or blue glass could accelerate or relax the nervous system to achieve balance within the body. One year later in 1878, Dr. Edwin Babbitt in his classic, *The Principles of Light and Color* described devices that utilized colored filters with both natural and artificial light to treat people. His Chromo Disk, fitted with specific filters, could be focused on specific areas of the body for treatment. He also developed solar elixirs by irradiating water with sunlight and then filtering it through a special Chromo Lens. (69)

It was during this same twenty-year span (1880-1900) that it was discovered that many specific bacteria were sensitive to ultraviolet light. Thus it was that ultraviolet light came to be used as a disinfectant in health care facilities and as a treatment for certain injuries and infections. (70)

Also in the 1890's it was discovered that rickets could be cured by sunlight, but why this was so, was not known until a further discovery that sunlight striking the skin produced vitamin D3, which is a necessary ingredient for the absorption of calcium and other minerals from the diet that are essential for normal growth and development of bones. D3 is really a hormone called cholecalciferol and is produced by the body in response to ultraviolet radiation. This is *not* the same vitamin D found in dairy products or vitamin tablets. It has never been found to be toxic while commercially manufactured vitamin D2 can be at high levels. (70-71)

Other pioneers like Niels Finsen, Dinshah Ghadiali, and Dr. Harry Spitler made significant findings in the 1890's. Niels Finsen, the "father of photobiology," successfully treated skin tubercular lesions with ultraviolet light, and used red light to prevent scar formation from smallpox. (71) Dinshah Ghadiali began the science of Spectro-Chrome, utilizing his extensive background in physics, chemistry, mathematics, and electricity. Spectro-Chrome is a precise scientific approach to the application of color to various parts of the human body. It is based on several scientific findings/intuitive assumptions:

1. Every chemical element in an excited state gives off "a distinctive set of
   colored bands called spectral emission lines" known as Fraunhofer lines.

2. When exposed to white light, the excited element will absorb the same frequencies that it gives off.

3. The major color emitted by an element of the body (i.e. heart)

is related to that element's function in the body.

4.   When used therapeutically, this color would aid the activity of this element in the body. [17]

Although not yet scientifically validated, Liberman relates the testimony of Dr. Kate Baldwin, senior surgeon at Philadelphia Woman's Hospital for twenty-three years, when she reported at a meeting of the Pennsylvania Medical Society in 1926 that (with regard to the action of colors in restoring body functions)

> I can produce quicker and more accurate results with colors than with any or all other methods combined—and with less strain on the patient...Septic conditions yield, regardless of the specific organism. Cardiac lesions, asthma, hay fever, pneumonia, inflammatory conditions of the eyes, corneal ulcers, glaucoma, and cataracts are relieved by the treatment.[18]

While Dinshah was developing the Spectro-Chrome system, Dr. Harry Spitler was researching and clinically using light therapy techniques. His observations led him to trying light therapy through the eyes. As a result of several years of trial in the 1920's, Spitler concluded that "although heredity, environment, and nutrition, play major roles in our lives, light may play the most significant role in altering function, behavior, and physiological response; in other words, merely altering the color of light entering the eyes can disturb or restore balance within the autonomic nervous system and thus effect resultant functions." [19]

Spitler went on to developing instruments that would shine various colors on the eyes. Liberman writes that Spitler believed that "light therapy by way of the eyes could augment the major control centers in the brain that regulate all body functions." [20]

Based on these findings/assumptions, Dr. Harry Spitler

conceived of a new science called Syntonics. He founded the College of Syntonic Optometry in 1933 that continues today as a post-doctoral educational optometric organization in the field of ocular phototherapy.

About The College of Syntonic Optometry and Syntonics

The College of Syntonic Optometry is an active and growing post-graduate educational organization with branches in Australia, Europe, Mexico, and Great Britain. Established in 1933, its members include optometrists and other health professionals and supporters from around the world. Those who achieve a clinical level of experience and mastery are awarded the status of Fellow.

The annual CONFERENCE ON LIGHT AND VISION features basic and advanced courses in syntonic phototherapy as well as presentations by scientists and clinicians from related fields.

It publishes THE JOURNAL OF OPTOMETRIC PHOTOTHERAPY as well as periodic newsletter updated and this website and others.

Today, scientific as well as clinical verification of light's impact on health and healing and a growing public demand for functional and rehabilitative vision therapy continue to vitalize the college and advance its mission.

Syntonics or optometric phototherapy, is the branch of ocular science dealing with the application of selected light frequencies through the eyes. It has been used clinically for over 70 years in the field of optometry with continued success in the treatment of visual dysfunctions, including strabismus (eye turns), amblyopia (lazy eye), focusing and convergence problems, learning disorders, and after effects of stress and trauma. In recent years, Syntonics has been shown to be effective in the treatment of brain injuries and emotional disorders.

Light is essential to life. Our planet revolves around the sun and all life on earth is sustained by sunlight. The Greeks were the first to document the use of phototherapy. Currently light is used on a variety of disorders from the "bili" lights used on jaundiced newborns to the more recent psychiatric use of white light for the treatment of Seasonal Affective Disorder (SAD). In optometry the use of phototherapy to treat visual dysfunctions is called Syntonics.

Interest in the effect of light on the body intensified earlier this century. Most of the current therapeutic techniques used in syntonics are based on the work done by Dr. Harry Riley Spitler in the 1920s and 1930s. Dr. Spitler, who had both optometric and medical degrees, began researching and using phototherapy in 1909. Spitler, the author of *The Syntonic Principle*, conceived the principles for a new science that he called "Syntonics". Syntonics, from the word syntony (to bring into balance) refers physiologically to a balanced integrated nervous system.

Certain biochemical conditions in the brain need to be present before effective cortical plasticity and new functions can occur. Neurotransmitters trigger this biochemistry and allow for additional synoptic connections to initiate movement and growth in new directions. Colored light therapy can act as a powerful tool to stimulate the biochemistry of the brain through the visual system by way of the retinal-hypothalamus brain connection.

A New Vision for Vision Specialists

The discovery of the successful treatment of bacterial infections with the first antibiotic, sulfanilamide, the "silver bullet" set the field of light therapy back into the field of witchcraft rather than of a non- intrusive miracle cure. Pharmaceutical companies pushed the new "wonder-drug" and it became the "magic pill" which would rid us of life threatening infections. Liberman laments, that we should have realized that it was our lifestyles, not bacteria, that caused disease. Our bodies are home to countless bacteria in balance within us. It is only when something occurs to create an imbalance that bacteria contribute to disease. (80)

Antibiotics have been a mixed blessing. Extensive use of them over time has had the same results on bacteria as pesticides have had on insects. Bacteria, in reaction to antibiotics, have become stronger. Highly resistant strains have evolved so that in the 2000s we find some strains that do not respond to antibiotics.

While the antibiotic evolution was in progress, Dr. T. A. Bromback, in 1936, found the "sixty-nine percent of children with diagnosed reading problems had a measurable enlargement in the portion of the optic nerve originating in the back of the eye." [21]

Bromback felt that the enlargement of this "blind spot" affected full visual perception and hence negatively affected reading ability. Over the next twenty years, Dr. Thomas Eames, a physician at Boston University, in a series of three studies, found that

1. Nine percent of the school children in these studies had constricted fields of vision, and of these nine percent, eighty- three percent were failing in schoolwork in one or more subjects.

2. Visual field constrictions significantly limited the speed of visual perceptions: and

3. Children with learning disabilities consistently had smaller visual fields than children without learning disabilities. [22, 23]

Were these conditions the cause or the result of academic

stress? Liberman and Virginia I. Shipman feel that stress causes a person to observe, see, remember, and learn less. [24]

Our fields of vision not only indicate how much of the whole picture we are seeing, but also how much of our brain is functioning. Under very demanding and stressful conditions such as schoolwork, our field of vision contracts and we become near sighted, as forty-five percent of the total United States population is. Clinical experience with Syntonics (color therapy through the eyes) resulted in expanded visual-field-size, and improvement in other visual functions as well. Liberman cites a number of case studies indicating the positive effects of Syntonics on learning disabilities, glaucoma, stroke rehabilitation, and retinitis pigmentosa (defective night vision). He doesn't claim that light therapy would be effective in *all* cases involving the aforementioned problems, but that since this therapy has been effective in a number of such cases, we should not close our minds as to what conditions are treatable with light therapy.

Light, Color and Learning

It is a fact that for the sighted person, most learning occurs visually and that the eyes are the *major* entryway for light into the body. Since this is the case, what effect, if any, would modifying the general lighting and/or environmental color have in the school environment? In this chapter, Liberman cites the work of Dr. Harry Wohlfarth, Barbara M. Vitale, and Dr. Helen Irlen.

In 1981 Dr. Harry Wohlfarth and his associate Catherine Sam conducted the first of his experimental studies designed to evaluate "the combined impact of selected colors and full-spectrum lighting on the behavior and physiology of both blind children with severe behavioral disorders and sighted children with severe handicaps" (101).

The monitoring and measuring of both physiology and

40

behavior took place both before and after full-spectrum lighting was installed and classroom walls painted with selected shades of warm colors (yellow and orange). The results were:

1. In experimental rooms, systolic blood pressure dropped an average twenty points per child.

2. Aggressive behavior and other forms of misbehavior dramatically reduced.

3. When room lighting changed back to cool-white florescent tubes, blood pressure increased as did incidents of disorderly behavior.

4. Blind subjects were affected as sighted ones (101-102)

In a second study conducted during the 1982-1983 school year using four similarly matched elementary schools, Wohlfarth evaluated more variables simultaneously than had previously been studied. "The purpose of the study was to evaluate the effects of different environmental light and/or color conditions on systolic blood pressure, mood states, absences due to illness, total disciplinary incidences, classroom noise levels, I.Q. test scores, and academic performance over a full year of school" (102).

Results:

School #1 – (Cool white fluorescents and left in original condition)...worst results.

School #2 – (Lighting and wall colors changed)best results for all areas except discipline. Students less stressed, quieter, less moody, great improvement on combined academic and I.Q. test scores, absences due to illness only one-third as often as School #1. Full spectrum lights and warm shades of light yellow and light blue wall paint.

41

School #3 – (Only lighting changed- retained original wall colors of orange, white, beige brown)no significant differences reported.

School #4 – (Only wall colors changed) had lowest disciplinary incidences.

With such impressive results Liberman wonders, "why all children's classrooms are not designed with such warm colors and full-spectrum lighting" (102-103).

Barbara Miester Vitale (*Unicorns Are Real: A Right Brained Approach to Learning*, and *Free Flight: Celebrating Your Right Brain*) has experimented with color in her work as educator since 1970. She reported in a letter to Liberman such interesting observations as:

1. The color red seems to be the most effective for reducing activity levels;

2. Children experience an increase in long term recall when notes are taken in their favorite color;

3. Some adults and children respond very well to reading or working under blue light, and

4. The value of color seems to be individual specific. In most cases, the color that works most effectively is either the person's favorite color or the color that is opposite on the color wheel. (103-104)

Dr. Helen Irlen, a California psychologist, became a national celebrity when her work was featured on a May 15, 1988 segment of "60 Minutes" called "Reading by Colors." By using client selected tinted lenses she transformed non reading, learning-disabled individuals into fluent readers while people watched. Not a new approach—one that has been used by the College of Syntonic Optometry for fifty-eight years. The problem with her method of treatment is that persons who wear the specific color tinted lenses all during their waking hours are placing themselves on a limited spectrum diet which can cause other problems. (104-105)

Light: Nature's Miracle Medicine

From ancient times people have recognized that cyclic or rhythmic patterns are an integral part of the functioning of all systems. In fact, these patterns are the basis for scientific predictions whose accuracy is contingent upon the assumption of orderly repetitiveness. Liberman asserts that this orderliness is "probably outside our universe" but eventually affects the tiniest atomic particle: from the universe to solar system—to earth—to the climate, seasons, inhabitants—to the tiniest atomic particle. (119)

The observation of these orderly patterns was and is used by many philosophers to "prove" the existence of a divine being, who established and constantly guides this orderliness. If this is so, then the well being of all living things is directly related to their openness to live in harmony with this orderliness, because we cannot escape the process!

Liberman poses two questions, the answers to which will help us to better understand the interrelatedness of human life and environment cycles. (119)

1. What do the seasons describe?
    That *all* living things have specific daily and seasonal rhythms. Seasonal changes provoke certain physiological and emotional changes within animals and humans. (119-120)

2. How does the activity of each season affect our lives during

that season?

a. *Spring*: a time for awakening, new beginnings, spring-cleaning, new life;

b. *Summer*: a time to grow and mature, to fulfill, summer camp get-away- from-it-all time;

c. *Fall*: slow walks amid the burst of colors around us (temperate zones), maturity on the verge of decline; and

d. *Winter*: a time of coldness (temperate zones) and stillness, clearing off the old and getting ready for a fresh start.

Spring and summer stimulate activity and growth of all sorts— externalization, while fall and winter are times for gradually living inside more—in our homes and in our innermost beings. (120)

Winter is meant to be a time for quiet introspection, taking stock of ourselves so to speak. But for many persons it is a time of sadness and depression because they are affected with a disorder called "Seasonal Affective Disorder" (SAD). Research has shown that persons living in northern climates are three times as likely to be affected by this disorder versus those living in southern climates.

The tendency to stay indoors and out of natural daylight for prolonged periods has been found to be the common cause, and exposure to full spectrum light, of a certain intensity, and for a certain duration, has "significant antidepressant effects on more than eighty-percent of those suffering from SAD" (124).

Non-seasonal depressions also seem to respond to full spectrum light therapy. Rae cites the experience of Daniel Kripke, M.D., professor of psychiatry at the University of California at San Diego. Since 1981, Dr. Kripke has been using light therapy on patients hospitalized for depression.

Kripke states that, "The benefit we are seeing is actually more than you would expect to see with antidepressant drugs in a comparable time period." [25]

Like Liberman, Kripke believes that the light therapy has this effect by affecting the melatonin levels in the body. Melatonin is the hormone secreted by the pineal gland located deep in the brain's core. The pineal gland "is the body's light meter and timer, orchestrating our internal functions and synchronizing them with the external environment of nature." [26] If the internal clock of humans is awry, it is probably because our living habits deprive too many of us of the natural light we need to make our pineal glands function as they should. The intensity and duration of the natural light to which we are daily exposed directly affect the amount of melatonin secreted by the pineal gland. The level of this hormone in our bloodstream affects our sexual functioning, sleep patterns, and mood changes. Higher levels of melatonin are secreted at night and lower levels during natural daylight. High levels depress sexual physiology, that is, decreased sex hormone levels, slow sexual maturation. Jet lag and altered sleep patterns also respond positively to carefully timed exposure to natural light.

Charles A. Czeisler, Ph.D., M.D., director of the Laboratory for Circadian and Sleep Disorders Medicine at Harvard Medical School and Brigham and Women's Hospital, was part of a team that discovered that light therapy could help astronauts reset their body clocks if they were working odd hours or expected to launch late at night. His work with astronauts led to a simple light treatment for jet lag. Spend parts of the next two days outdoors in natural light—to be synchronized to local time with the coming of dawn on the third day. That's it! A similar procedure has helped older persons who need or want to stay up past their ever-diminishing "sleepy time." They are simply exposed to bright light in the early evening to delay their sleep-wake cycles. [27]

Full-spectrum light, is also being used in Dentistry and

Acupuncture. In Dentistry, as I experienced, a beam of light is being used to "cure" a photo active composite material used in fillings, which more nearly resembles the natural color of teeth. In Acupuncture, Russian scientists have been experimenting with laser puncture that utilizes low-energy laser beams rather than needles to stimulate acupuncture points.

Could many rhythmic disorders be merely cues to point out to us how out of touch we are with our bodies and with nature in general? Are at least some of these conditions we've just examined really medical disorders or rather symptoms of something deeper that we don't understand? [28]

Liberman writes that many popular medical applications of light therapy are treating symptoms rather than causes. It is time to take a more holistic approach—an approach that looks at all aspects of a person: mind, body, emotions, and spirit. Perhaps it's time we started looking within ourselves for answers rather than constantly treating ourselves as the victims of some strange new disease. (135- 136)

UV or Not UV: That Is the Question

Be cautious! Stay out of the sun. Protect yourself from exposure to *all* Ultraviolet light by using sun-blocking sunglasses, protective clothing, and sun block lotions at SPF 25 and 30.

These warnings are everywhere in the media and advertising. What are the real facts about sunlight?

It is generally agreed in scientific circles that ultraviolet light in *large* amounts is harmful, but according to Liberman, John Ott, and others, in *trace* amounts, as in natural light, ultraviolet light acts as a "life-supporting nutrient" (140).

There are three different classifications of ultraviolet light according to wavelength:

1. Near-Ultraviolet (UV-A) (320-380 nanometers), directly adjoining the violet end of the visible-light spectrum—responsible for the tanning response in humans.

2. Mid-Ultraviolet (UV-B) (290-320 nanometers), appears to activate the synthesis of Vitamin D and the absorption of calcium and other minerals from the diet. R.M. Neer's study in 1971 concluded that the group of elderly veterans receiving UV-B absorbed forty percent more calcium than their counterparts who received no ultraviolet exposure. [29]

3. Far-Ultraviolet (UV-C) (100-290 nanometers), mostly filtered out by the Earth's ozone layer, is germicidal, killing bacteria, viruses, and other infectious agents. [30]

Other benefits of Ultraviolet light claimed by studies cited in Liberman do not specify which classification of ultraviolet light used in terms of A, B, or C. Some of the benefits claimed are:

1. Ultraviolet light lowers blood pressure. (J.R. Johnson, "The Effects of Carbon Arc Radiation on Blood Pressure and Cardiac Output," *American Journal of Physiology* 114 (1935): p. 594).

2. Ultraviolet light increases the efficiency of the heart (becomes stronger and pumped more blood)—thirty-nine per- cent increase in eighteen of the twenty persons tested. (Same study as in #1)

3. Ultraviolet light reduces cholesterol. Ninety-seven percent of patients with hypertension and other circulatory problems, two hours after exposure to ultraviolet light had a thirteen percent decrease in serum cholesterol levels. Eighty- six percent maintained this level twenty-four hours later. (R. Atlschul and I. H. Herman, *Ultraviolet Irradiation and Cholesterol*

Metabolism; Seventh Annual Meeting of the American Society for the Study of Arteriosclerosis, Circulation 8 (1953): p. 438). (142)

4. Ultraviolet light is an effective treatment for psoriasis for up to eighty percent of sufferers. (L. Lohmerer, "Let The Sun Shine In," *East West*, July 1986, pp. 36-39).

5. Ultraviolet light is an effective treatment for many other diseases among which are several forms of tuberculosis bacteria, black lung disease, and severe asthma. Several Russian and German studies confirm this use. (143)

6. Ultraviolet light activates an important skin hormone, solitrol, believed to be a form of vitamin D3 which influences many of the body's regulatory centers as well as the immune system. (144)

Other benefits are cited for *proper* use of ultraviolet light. It is exposure to inordinate amounts of ultraviolet light that causes problems. Trace amounts of ultraviolet light are as vital to human health as are trace amounts of other vital nutrients.

Many persons are experiencing health problems due to a lack of proper lighting in the environments where they live and work. Normal daily summer days shine with up to 100,000 lux while the typical indoor environment is 600-700 lux. In addition the commonest form of home lighting, the incandescent lamp bulb, gives off practically no ultraviolet light and concentrates most of its light energy in the yellow, red, and infrared portions of the spectrum. Sunlight, on the other hand, contains the entire spectrum peaking in the blue-green area of the visible spectrum.

Fluorescent tubes emit a small amount of ultraviolet light which is usually shielded/ absorbed. They also give off mercury vapor, in levels, according to Ott, that are much higher than admitted, as well as x-rays and radio wave emissions. Ott feels that the deluxe warm-white fluorescent and the cool white ones, because of their limited and harmful spectrums, should be absolutely avoided. (146-147)

The studies done on animals with ultraviolet light are flawed because they all exposed animals to highly abnormal amounts of ultraviolet light in unnatural ways. For example, the monkeys used in one experiment had their eyelids clamped open and a 2,500 watt xenon lamp beamed high levels of ultraviolet light into their exposed eyes for sixteen minutes. This would never happen in real life so how are the results generalizable to *normal* exposure sunlight? (W. T. Ham, et.al., "Action Spectrum For Retinal Injury From *Near Ultraviolet* Radiation in the Aphakic Monkey," *American Journal of Ophthalmology* (March 1982). Also how does this research relate to humans?

Liberman asks whether, in fact, we are creating our own blindness by wearing sunglasses that block out *all* ultraviolet light. He cites an article by John Marshall of the University of London, entitled "Light and the Ageing Eye" in which Marshall states that the body is made up of two different cell systems, one of which constantly renews itself by dividing (cornea, skin, etc.), and the other does not (brain, retina, etc.). Marshall cites as an example of a lifelong non-dividing cell, the pigment epithelium cells of the retina. These cells become diseased as a result of absorbing an excess amount of ultraviolet light over a lifetime.

While studying the pigment epithelium cells of a rabbit's eye, "Ott noticed that the colors of filters used to view the cells significantly affected the biological responses within the cells themselves. Further, Ott noticed that these cells would divide *only if low levels of ultraviolet radiation were projected into them*" (149).

So, pigment epithelium cells *do* divide in the presence of ultraviolet light. That John Marshall was incorrect may be due to the fact that the light source of the microscope he used did not contain ultraviolet radiation! (149) If Ott is correct, then our typical lifestyle, which seeks to block out all ultraviolet light, may be resulting in certain degenerative eye conditions.

Our beliefs on the causative relationship between exposure to ultraviolet light and the incidence of skin cancer are also challenged by Liberman. He relates the published facts regarding ultraviolet radiation and cancer: parts of the body most commonly exposed most likely to get skin cancer, lighter skinned persons who get sunburned repeatedly are likely cancer candidates as are people who live in tropical and subtropical latitudes. (150) But there was a study done by Dr. Helen Shaw and published in the August 7, 1982 British medical journal *Lancet,* which claimed that the incidence of malignant melanomas was considerably higher in office workers who worked all day under fluorescent lights than in persons *regularly* exposed to sunlight due to their lifestyle or occupation.

Two other carefully controlled studies conducted at the New York University School of Medicine confirmed Shaw's findings.

The only clear thing with regard to ultraviolet exposure and skin cancer is that over exposure and certain skin types are major cancer risk factors. Moderate sensible exposure is both safe and desirable. Many other factors (nutrition, lifestyle, etc.,) need to be evaluated for how else do we account for the near absence of cancer among many persons who live at high altitudes or near the equator where the ultraviolet exposure is high? (151)

Liberman makes some final recommendations regarding sunlight exposure. Spend a portion (at least one hour) outdoors each day, regardless of weather. Don't wear sunglasses, prescription glasses, contacts or sun tan lotion unless it is an extremely sunny day that feels too bright. Avoid exposure between the hours of 10:00 a.m. and 2:00 p.m. If you must wear sunglasses, wear neutral gray ones that reduce the entire spectrum in a balanced way. Don't use sun tan lotion with PASA—can be carcinogenic in the sun. Build up time in the sun gradually—use no sun tan lotion at all if you have moderate to dark skin. (153)

Have we gone too far in our attempt to blot out exposure to all ultraviolet light even though it is necessary to our health in trace amounts? Dr. Zane Kime thinks so: "The most 'biologically active' part of sunlight is the ultraviolet. It is absolutely critical for optimal health." [31]

Getting Well with the Rainbow Diet

Our entire blood supply circulates through our eyes about every two hours. Parts of the eye like the aqueous humor, lens, and vitreous humor, act as windows that allow light to directly stimulate the eyes and blood and to indirectly stimulate all other bodily functions…"every substance (vitamin, mineral, chemical, etc.,) ingested by the body as food has a *maximum wavelength absorption characteristic*…for any ingested substance to be fully processed or used by the body, it needs to go through a series of chemical reactions that are catalyzed (ignited) by a specific portion of the electromagnetic spectrum" (157-158).

Liberman claims that most foods are light in solid form. How nutritional our food is depends on how low on the food chain it is. Things lowest on the food chain (vegetables, fruits, grains, etc.) are made directly from light through the process of photosynthesis. The color of the food we eat also reveals aspects of its nutritional content, like which of the body's major energy centers (the chakras), located approximately at the sites of the major endocrine glands, it is meant to nourish.

Dr. Gabriel Cousins, author of *Spiritual Nutrition and the Rainbow Diet*, writes that the color of food in addition to indicating the specific endocrine area of the body it is meant to nourish, also indicates the time of day we should eat this

51

color food. We can eat white foods (full spectrum) any time during the day. Red, orange, and yellow, are the colors of sunrise so these colors of foods are "beginning the day" foods, green is a midday (luncheon) food color, while blue, indigo, and violet and golden grains are sunset and evening (dinner) foods. (159-160)

Cousins diet is vegetarian because these are all lower chain (closer to light) foods, while meat, fish, etc., are higher chain, more remote from light, foods. Irradiated or over processed foods are nutritionally dead, having lost their light energy in the processing.

A New Paradigm for Health and Healing

The last three chapters of Liberman's are futuristic in outlook. He entitles this part of his book "Light Years Beyond." In Chapter Thirteen, the first of these futuristic chapters, Liberman describes what he calls "a new Paradigm for Health and Healing."

It isn't germs and viruses that cause diseases, it is our lifestyles, the way we respond to stress, etc., that opens the door to imbalance and disease. Instead of focusing on killing microorganisms (like with antibiotics) we would be better off starving the offending microorganisms by changing our mental, emotional, and physical environments that *feed* these organisms. We need to concentrate our healing efforts on locating and dealing with the *causes* of our problems and not just on their effects. We need to deal with deep inner healing. (165-166)

Liberman maintains that the successful doctor must be much more than a master technician. He/she must be able to personally relate to their patients' situations because, "good techniques will always follow, rather than lead, the healing process" (168).

The successful healer must have worked through his/her own pain first and come to terms with it, before he/she can effectively heal others. Liberman describes his own personal journey through pain and insecurity. The process he went through is called "Focusing" though he doesn't use that term.

Liberman, like most of us, daily faced all the pain and insecurities of his past life. If he "focused" on the pain long enough, that is, just to be present to it—allow himself to be with it, something welled up from deep within him that allowed him to accept his pain, to be patient with himself. He relates that this "intuitive wisdom" was all the smartness he needed to work with himself and others. (172)

Focusing, a therapeutic method developed by Eugene Gendlin of the University of Chicago, which I mentioned earlier in this Chapter, is a way to bring to consciousness the body's wisdom. It requires quiet and patience as Liberman asserts. One has to learn how to come out of head thinking into body awareness, how something feels in one's body, particularly in the "gut" or solar plexus. It is a discipline of attending to the bodily "felt-sense" of what is at work in one's life – our fears and our insecurities, etc. It is a way of being present to these things in a caring loving way. It is a method that enables us to contact our inner vulnerability and repressed pain and in so doing release new energy and new hope that lead us to being able to understand and live with our pain and imperfections.

Edwin M. McMahon and Peter A. Campbell, in their book, *Bio-Spirituality*, which describes Focusing as a way for the whole person to grow, include spirituality, as the essential part of the self-discovery process. They identify three basic experiences that Focusing can help one enter and learn *the truth of themselves.* These three experiences are:

1. Fear of losing control vs. the risk of letting go and allowing.

2. New identity in being gifted, led, graced, and

3. Bodily felt meaning as key to spiritual growth (that growth is grounded in a deep knowledge of what is deepest in the feelings, the very being of one's self).[32]

Liberman believes that our total life experiences, physiological, psychological, and spiritual are simply different energy frequencies that can be measured in terms of EKG and EEGs. Our bodies, as Teilhard de Chardin would agree, are highly complex organisms. Liberman calls them "radar screens" that receive, record, and transmit these energies. These energies collectively equal "experience." [33]

In addition to all of the energies associated with physiological functions there is the energy transmitted by the body as light, specifically as various portions of the spectrum. Fritz Albert Popp reported in *Brain/Mind Bulletin* 10, #14 (August 19, 1985) that cells of living things radiate "biophotons" ranging the entire electromagnetic spectrum. Their intensity varies according to the specific biochemical reaction taking place. (173)

Liberman cites the finding of Indian scientists and physicians that the electromagnetic fields surrounding living things can by the specific color they give off, predict/identify disorders ranging from brain tumors to schizophrenia. (174)

All the energy involved in these transactions is in a state of constant change. Liberman would agree with the Greek philosopher Democritus who maintained that everything was in such constant and rapid process of change that it was impossible to place our feet in the same stream twice. The water had moved on. John Dewey, the pragmatist father of American public school education, believed that the ultimate in the universe was not "being," but "process." Change was at the very heart of things, and scientific method was the way we could understand and cope with this constant on-goingness.

Our bodies are sieve like receptors through which energy

(basically light) flows. When this flow is cut off or blocked for some reason, part of us malfunctions. If we can find the specific portion of the spectrum that the malfunctioning radiates, and expose the body to that same portion of the spectrum, the blockage is opened and the flow of light resumes.

"State of mind determines energy assimilation, which, over time, alters brain circuitry patterns and eventually determines the state of health" (177). Once again, treatment with the appropriate portion of the spectrum can restore balance that is needed.

We are the products of heredity and environment. Our life's experiences begin even before birth and accumulate to make us what we are at each stage of our earth lives. Early traumas cause us to be unreceptive or allergic both emotionally and psychologically to aspects of some of our experiences—we bury them deep within ourselves and try to keep them there. We avoid people and circumstances that trigger these painful problems. As McMahon and Campbell assert in *Bio-Spirituality* through Focusing, deep healing occurs when through an internal bodily felt process, "we are able to befriend what is disturbing us and thereby free ourselves from our hurtful allergic reaction to them" (177).

To Liberman true healing is a process called...Homeopathy. It begins within us and then affects not only the within but also the without, our bodies. It treats the whole person. (179)

The modern concept of homeopathy was developed by Dr. Samuel Hahnemann in 1810. It rests on the "Law of Similars" (Hippocrates and Paracelsus): "Let likes be treated by likes." In other words, "the most appropriate remedy for a patient is one with a *vibration* that is *equivalent* to the patient's pathology." The work of Royal Raymond Rife (1888-1971) which I presented under the examination of Chapter Nine of Liberman's book, advocates precisely this form of treatment.

Various viruses, which Rife listed, glow with specific colors according to type of virus. By irradiating these pathogenic organisms with specific frequencies (MORs) he caused them to devitalize, either by interrupting their normal cytologic function or by inducing them to mutate into a non-pathogenic form.[34] "Let likes be treated by likes."

The basic principles of homeopathy and of Bio-Spirituality are very similar. Both speak of the interconnectedness of the mind and body. In fact, the human person is spoken of as a mind-body complex in which, during this earth life at least, the union of the two is so profound that one part simply does not function well (and mostly not at all) without the other. With every passing year, the medical research builds, that supports the interconnectedness of mental and physical disorders. Both homeopathy and Bio-Spirituality also stress that in the process of healing, deep emotional issues often must be dealt with *first* and then their physical counterparts. Finally, although many aspects of human behavior, personality, and appearance, are learned coping mechanisms, many are also deeply rooted in our personality/physical type and thus produce non-thinking reflex type reactions to various stimuli in our environments.

The Enneagram, originally developed by the Sufis and brought into modern times by various psychologists and Christian therapists, lists nine different personality types with their corresponding behaviors. By studying the Enneagram we can discern our own basic personality type and better understand why we behave the way we do. We can learn healthy, whole person ways, of allowing us to accept ourselves as we are, and be able to act in loving giving/affirming ways. Helen Palmer's *The Enneagram in Love and Work*, and Peter Hannan's *Nine Faces of God* provide an excellent understanding of the Enneagram and its application to every aspect of our lives.

Gentleness in dealing with ourselves and with each other, is the key to the deepest healing.

Liberman states, that the life experiences that arouse our feelings bring us to an awareness of what is really hurting us. We box in those things and hide the things that we most need. St. Paul says the same thing in "religious language": "We groan in pain as we await the redemption of our bodies." We have to be willing to deal with the most painful aspects of our lives in caring, loving ways, and allow the life force deep within to heal us. [35]

Becoming Illuminated With Light

Thus, Liberman sets the scope for this chapter by reemphasizing that light is the basic tool needed to treat both the "within" (our emotional and mental states), and also the "without" (our functions and pathologies). (183)

He goes on to relate what he was taught in syntonics and how his experience with this light therapy caused him to develop new methods. He found that Spitler's original model of syntonics based on medical theories of the 1920's viewed the basis for dysfunctions and diseases primarily as the result of psychological imbalances rather than emotional ones. Liberman's book would demonstrate the opposite—emotional issues were primary and led to the imbalance that made the body vulnerable to dysfunction/disease.

Although the treatment seemed simplistic to him, it worked. But Liberman wanted to go deeper. He wanted to know the underlying issues at the root of dysfunctions. He also wanted to look at how he was dealing with traumatic feelings in his own life. (184-185)

If one really wants to get rid of weeds he has to *completely* uproot them. The same is true for deep lasting healing to take place. As painful and time consuming at it is we have to be willing to surface (that is, bring to consciousness) deeply imbedded issues because the subconscious is responsible for up to ninety percent of who we are and how we function. Liberman and Focusing therapy align once more.

We need to first allow whatever is bothering us to surface, be with these issues gently and friendly, and then rebond with our innermost "gut level" feelings, our hearts. This entire process will affect all our "functioning and being" (186).

Dealing with our emotions, our feelings, is the first step to lasting healing. Liberman discovered that the so-called "rules" (question #2) about the effects of various filters varied according to the person involved. Magenta, for example, calmed some and disturbed others. He also found that, as painful and time consuming as it may be, reconnecting with the original underlying causes of the disturbance was a prerequisite to emotional healing.

Individual differences in the receptivity to specific colors was directly related to past experiences (traumas or beneficent) in patients' lives. At this point, Liberman mentions the work of Royal R. Rife and his (Rife's) findings, that irradiating the cancerous organism with the same color light it gave off would destroy the organism.

Liberman also writes of the relationship between light and addictive behavior. He noticed in his therapy sessions with alcoholics that addictive personalities became more or less addictive depending on the colors at which they looked—the colors the individual was *most* uncomfortable with led to the strongest urges for alcohol. As he had increasing experiences with addictive patients he came to realize more and more that situations that triggered a significant level of fear/discomfort with which we were unable to be present (that is, allow in our consciousness) caused us to seek escape in addictive behavior. (188)

It is once more a matter of bodily knowing rather than conscious decision making. "The body may know that the energy content of a particular food/drink…vodka, when combined with the energy content of fear may temporarily alleviate that fear. *This I believe is the basis for all addiction*" (Italicizing is mine) (188).

Gentleness and loving concern on the part of a therapist is essential for healing a patient. Treating a patient with color therapy by way of their eyes stimulates patients to express the old and unresolved emotional issues that were behind the physical dysfunctioning. The therapist becomes a loving, caring, listening presence.

It is interesting to note that the colors with which people were most uncomfortable "correlated almost one hundred percent of the time with the portions of their bodies (chakra chart) where they housed stress, developed disease, or had injured themselves." Once these painful issues had been addressed, these same colors that had stimulated discomfort now brought joy and euphoria. (189-190)

Light: The Final Frontier

Liberman writes that, "Light is the superterrestrial, natural force under which all life on Earth originates and develops" (203). I would agree and add "Light is also *the* Supernatural Force (*above* and *before* nature). For Christians, Light centered in three Persons constituting one Divine Being is God.

Light therapy is a non-invasive technology unlike the commonest therapies of today, which involve powerful very invasive drugs with all kinds of undesirable side effects. At times it is a toss- up as to which is worse, the proposed cure or the disease! We are into the "light age." If Liberman is accurate in his predictions, "Scalpels will be replaced by lasers, chemotherapy by phototherapy, prescription drugs by prescription colors, acupuncture needles by needles of light, eye glasses by healthy eyes. Cancer will be a disease of the past" (205).

As noted previously, light therapy deals with the intimate relationship between body and mind (spirit). The affective (emotional) side of us is seen as foundation in terms of physical health. Present traditional analysis, counseling, and medication, often concentrate on simply erasing the pain rather than finding its cause and dealing with it. They will be replaced by light therapy that sees and treats the mind *and* body as mind-body, one intimately connected, functioning, whole, system. The focus of light therapy is upon the person—the whole person and not on the disease.

Liberman concludes his book with two important statements: "The study of light affirms the interconnectedness of all things" and "Let the light in" (207)!

Since the publication of Jacob Liberman's book and the other work done by persons like David Tumey and William Sheline, improvements continued in the technology needed to deliver ever more efficient healing through the use of light.

When I went to Dr. Earl Lizotte's office for my annual eye exam in June of 2002, I told him that I had been experiencing some difficulty with "seeing" with my present prescription and I asked him if he thought that I needed another series of light treatments to build upon the series I had had nine years previously.

In 1993 the series was given several times a week—mine was three times per week for eight weeks. The results of these twenty-four treatments were significant improvement in vision acuity (sharpness of sight) especially in my right "lazy" eye, and the end of this eye being crossed and focusing with my left eye. I had dramatically expanded range of vision in all directions, and night vision. I could see colors and objects on my countryside walks after dark. But, in 2002, Dr. Lizotte pointed out to me that a new Spectral Receptivity System had been developed by Universal Light Technology in Carbondale,

Colorado, that was more powerful than the projection system I was exposed to in 1993. This was the system he was now using and the sessions were best given once a week over a period of weeks. I received ten treatments using the new Spectral Receptivity Trainer. Once again my vision acuity and range of vision improved significantly and some night vision returned. But, I failed to do any maintenance treatments so in 2006 my vision acuity had begun to decline. I was examined by Dr. Lizotte in March. My range of vision was fine and my right eye that was crossed and focusing with the left eye had remained straight since 1993. I went through a new series of treatments primarily to improve acuity in my right eye. This time I will keep a maintenance schedule.

The new description of the System by the Colorado company that produces it states:

> After many years of research and development, a quantum leap in science and technology has now given birth to the Spectral Receptivity System. Conceived by a visionary scientist and creatively "imagineered" by ATOMIC of Houston, the new Spectral Receptivity System is destined to be the "tool of the future" for expanding human consciousness and receptivity. Incorporating state-of-the-art technology, innovative design, superior quality, and precise manufacturing, the "new" Spectral Receptivity System is the most sophisticated educational color projection system ever designed.

Of the "State-of-the-Art Features" listed, three caught my attention in particular:

1. Twenty spectroscopically evaluated, designed, and balanced color filters—spanning the entire visible spectrum.

2. Extremely efficient—greatly expanded viewing field with increased light output...

3. State-of-the-art holographic light sculpting diffuser— providing a custom designed viewing field—effective for

both individual and group experience.

As noted in the description of the Spectral Receptivity System, the physical act of seeing with our eyes is but the window to expand awareness and consciousness that affects our entire lives. As noted over and over in Chapters II, III, and IV of this book, Teilhard de Chardin, Zajonc, Liberman, and others have stressed the interconnectedness of the without (the body) and the within (the mind and every form of psychism or consciousness). The outer and inner lights are intimately related, each affecting the other.

During our earth lives we experience constant change. How present and receptive we are to what life offers us each day has a significant effect on our wellness.

Dr. Earl Lizotte attended a series of training seminars given by Dr. Jacob Liberman in Aspen, Colorado in September 1994. The topic during one of the sessions was "Light, Life, and Expanding Consciousness." He took notes and kept the handout on the topic that he shared with me in early July, 2002. The direct quotes and other thoughts addressed in the rest of this chapter are from Dr. Lizotte's notes, his discussions with me, and my analysis and reactions. In "Light, Life and Expanding Consciousness," we read that "Jesus, Buddha, Socrates, Lao Tzu, and many others have all said that being present is the master key to everything—health, wellness, clarity, bliss, and spiritual evolution." I would add that McMahon and Campbell's work on *Bio-spirituality* (through the technique known as "focusing") says exactly the same thing.

This idea of "presence" as expressed in Light, Life, and Expanding Consciousness seems to be almost synonymous with "instinct." The example given of observing the actions of animals living in nature and noting that these actions are always a timely and appropriate response to life—an unthinking response not tied to any concepts or ideas of "mind," suggests that their response is automatic and instinctual.

Humans rarely do this. For we humans to be present to life depends on our answer to the question, "Are we the one noticing, not the thinker?" If we recognize that we are the one noticing, not the thinker, then we can begin to live life moment by moment, and thus not interfere with life's natural tendency towards health and wellness on every level.

From a Christian perspective, if we try to live our lives in conformity with the gospel, if we try to keep our hearts open to the promptings of the Holy Spirit, then we can just notice the thoughts we have, because the thinker is the Spirit.

If our inner light is really darkness, our thoughts may also be darkness. To just be aware of those thoughts, to notice them, is certainly essential to being present to life moment by moment. But to dismiss the concepts of a formed and informed conscience certainly does not lead to health and wellness physically, emotionally, mentally, or spiritually.

I would agree with the notes on Dr. Liberman's lecture where they relate that, "our lives are always a reflection of our state of consciousness and presence. Our experiences are a mirror image of the way we live our lives." Living in each moment means that we accept (but may not like) what life is offering. We try to see our lives as a whole, to focus on the entire doughnut and not the hole.

We are reminded once again that modern quantum Physicists believe that everything we experience is vibratory in nature—all matter is frozen in light. Life is actually light energy that appears to be solid because of an illusion created by the mind. Without powerful microscopes some things appear to be "solid" which are really in a constant state of flux.

Colors are one of these illusory projections of the mind due to our visual interpretations, the way we see the different vibrations that make up our experience. Phototherapy utilizes the fact that "the colors we are attracted to are the vibrational equivalencies of our life experiences that we are receptive to—the aspects of life we say "yes" to.

The colors we don't like (supposedly), relate to unresolved, negative, past experiences—our attempts to protect ourselves from life. If it is true that the colors we are unreceptive to, are a key to our expansion and healing, then becoming receptive to what we are resisting creates expansion of our consciousness and wellness on every level.

Dr. Lizotte shared with me his experience regarding the phototherapy treatment of three women who all had negative reactions to the color orange. He found that all of them had been sexually molested when very young. After the final phototherapy session one of the women came in wearing bright orange and a big smile. She told him that she had conquered the suppression of the molestation, was now able to be present to it, and felt a great sense of release. He discussed these cases and their results with several psychotherapists and found that they too had gotten the same results as he had, given the same repression, and the color orange.

In early 2006, Dr. Lizotte informed me of an exciting new use of light therapy that he was directly involved with at the North East Research Institute in Holyoke, Massachusetts called NERI.

It is a special education school for adolescents who are so seriously disruptive that they cannot function in a regular classroom. The school's first task is to try to discover the factor(s) that seem to cause these students to be disruptive.

Eye testing revealed that a substantial majority of these young people had functioning vision disabilities such as poor eye tracking which effectively prevented them from learning to read.

Dr. Lizotte decided to utilize tracking exercises and

balancing, "physical therapy for the eyes," using the Spectral Receptivity Trainer as the bedrock procedure for getting the students' autonomic nervous systems in balance. The results as of early spring 2006 are impressive. After a range of twelve to twenty-four treatments, dependent on each student's disability level, the treated students' disruptive behavior declines to the point where they are able to be mainstreamed into a regular classroom and are able to learn to read.

The Institute hopes to build each student's diagnosis and treatment into their individualized educational plan so that financial costs and human costs will be drastically reduced with a positive benefit to each adolescent and to society.

A New Light on Cancer

Based on all the information presented thus far, Liberman writes that we must expand our vision regarding the purpose of light. It is much more than illumination for our environment. It is "potentially one of the most powerful disease-prevention tools at our disposal" (109).

In a "leading edge" paper written by engineer and inventor David Tumey and his associate, William Sheline, entitled "Royal Rife Revisited: Reconstruction of the Original Rife Ray Tube," the authors describe a fascinating piece of equipment and its related therapeutical uses.

Royal Raymond Rife (1888-1971) was an accomplished scientist and microbiologist who developed an optical microscope that could provide magnifications, and resolutions heretofore unheard of...The major difference between visible light and electron microscopy is that by its nature, electron microscopes destroy the microorganisms while viewing them. Rife's major advantage was that he could image living virus and other microorganisms and observe them in their natural state...

It is argued that Rife was the first person to empirically prove that virus and bacteria are pleomorphic forms. Pleomorphism is the phenomenon by which one distinct life form mutates into another. Rife basically classified pathogenic bacteria into ten individual groups. Rife demonstrated that any organism within its group could be transformed morphologically into any other organism within the ten groups by carefully altering the media (light) in which it was cultured. *Of course this discovery contradicts modern microbiology which teaches that a bacteria's morphology is fixed and Unchangeable.* [26] (Italicizing is mine)

Rife also discovered techniques for successfully culturing cancer virus. This virus he identified as BX and it was noted that the viruses refracted a purplish red color with a monochromatic beam under his microscope. In fact, Rife discovered that each organism depending on its state would refract unique spectra and have distinct coloration. By the late 1920's and early 1930's Rife had discovered that by irradiating these pathogenic microorganisms with specific frequencies known as MOR's for Mortal Oscillatory Rates, he could cause them to devitalize either by interrupting normal cytologic function or by inducing them to mutate into a non-pathogenic form.

The authors go on to relate how Rife developed his original list of MORs by manipulating the dial of an audio frequency generator until he discovered a frequency that had the ability to devitalize a particular organism. By the mid 1950's he had developed a list of fifteen frequencies and the fifteen viruses they devitalized. The viruses on the list included Tetanus, Treponema, Gonorrhea, Staphylococci, Pneumococci, Streptothrix, Streptococci, Typhoid bacteria, Typhoid virus, Bacillus Coli Rod Form, Bacillus Coli Virus, Tuberculosis Rod Form, Tuberculosis Virus, Sarcoma (all forms?), and Carcinoma (all forms?). [27] (The question marks are Stafford's).

Tumey and Sheline describe how they went about

reconstructing the Rife Ray Tube. In the conclusion of their paper they indicate that the next logical step might be to repeat the laboratory studies of Dr. Stafford and others whose work utilizing Rife's MOR list in treating the associated viruses resulted in some amazing results as reported in Stafford's paper, "Electromagnetic Field Therapy" (1963).

In the conclusion of his paper Dr. Stafford writes:

Having worked with the specifically related field modality for the past six years, I am convinced that there exists some effective force in this form of therapy. This modality seems to exert some modifying force on the animal and human body...

If Mr. Rife's theory is right, then a method must be developed to isolate the offending organism in each specific case and find the exact frequency which causes that organism to disintegrate. These facts should be determined before treating each patient in every instance. With data of this sort available for each specific case before treatment, more consistent results should be obtained. To date, we are merely using data developed by Mr. Rife years ago. We only can hope that we are approaching the critical resonant frequency of the suspected pathogen. This is a very blind and unscientific approach, admittedly. Perhaps with adequate research, these weaknesses may be overcome. (10-11)

With the recreation of the Rife Ray Tube by David Tumey and William Sheline, it is now possible to do exactly what Dr. Robert Stafford recommended.

Liberman describes a number of experiments done with full spectrum light and/or specifically selected colors. Studies done on mice that were bred to develop tumors, indicated that a pink light environment resulted in the earliest development of tumors while full spectrum light inhibited the development of tumors for a twenty percent longer period of time. Older cells are more at risk for accumulated DNA damage that precedes cancer. Experiments done on fish and paramecia using near-ultraviolet radiation indicated that the damaged cells not only repaired themselves but also reversed their aging. What if it is discovered that human cells have the same capabilities?

Since 1900 when scientists first noted that certain substances were damaging to living tissue when exposed to light, but were not toxic in the dark, it has been discovered that many of these substances belong to a family of light-activated chemicals called porphyrins

During World War II (1942) it was noted that if porphyrins were present in one's body, tumors would fluoresce under light, brilliant red under ultraviolet light. This discovery was built upon in 1973 when technology made photodynamic therapy possible. Scientists found that certain photosensitive chemicals selectively identify cancer cells under ultraviolet light and accumulate in these cells. Then, under red light, these chemicals destroy the cancer cells. [38]

As of the 1991 publication date of *Light-Medicine of the Future*, only Photofrin (DHE) has been FDA approved for human use. After injection with a prescribed amount of Photofrin, the patient has to wait for up to seventy-two hours in an environment free of direct sunlight or other bright lights so that some of the Photofrin which also collects in certain normal tissues (kidneys, liver, spleen, and pancreas) can be eliminated. The treatment is delivered to the site of the tumor by hair thin fiber optic tubes. The result is that within hours the cancer cells begin to die leaving *most* normal tissues unharmed. "Even in tissues that are just partially cancerous, only the cancerous portions of the tissue will die. Since the specific photosensitive dyes are combined with highly tuned laser light, the treatment is extremely precise" (113).

In the February - March 1994 issue of *Modern Maturity* magazine, there is an article entitled "Bright Light, Big Therapy" by Stephen Rae. The article discusses light therapy's use in several areas such as overcoming jet lag, disturbed sleep, seasonal affective disorder, non-seasonal depressions, and a process called Photopheresis.

The Photopheresis process begins with an injection of Psoralen, a light sensitive substance made from a Nile River weed that is activated by ultraviolet light. The seventy year old patient described in the article was suffering from T-cell lymphoma, a cancer of the immune system in which certain white (T) blood cells "proliferated wildly, eventually overrunning the body and causing death within three or four years." [39]

An hour *after* the injection, the patient is attached by a tube in his arm to a blood cleansing machine which removes his blood, spins it to separate out the T-cells from the healthy red ones. The T-cells are then routed through a field of ultraviolet light that causes the Psoralen to crosslink their DNA and impede their ability to reproduce. Then the healthy and the irradiated sick T-cells are reinfused into the patient. Once back in the body it seems that Psoralen also modifies the T-cells structure so that they stimulate the immune system that then attacks both treated and untreated malignant cells. Francis Gasparro, a research scientist at Yale Medical School says that twenty-five percent of those treated remain symptom free five years after treatment and another fifty percent show some improvement. (84)

Liberman writes that this Photodynamic therapy, as of 1991, was being evaluated in approximately seventy different centers worldwide, forty-five of them in the United States and Canada.

New applications for this therapy include removing cholesterol from arteries and the decontamination of blood for transfusions. "Using the same photosensitive chemical (photofrin) and red light... researchers have been able to kill one-hundred percent of viruses causing herpes simplex type 1 (cold sores), measles, Aids, and other illnesses, without any evidence of damage to normal blood elements."

The next step beyond the non-laser regular light source used by Matthews will probably be special tunable lasers which were being used by scientists (1991) in the United States Governments' Strategic Defense Initiative (SDI) program. [40]

While working on this chapter of *Light-Medicine of the Future*, I had a dental appointment for a filling restoration. My dentist proceeded as usual in preparing the site and then packed the cavity with what I thought was the usual restorative material. Then I noticed that he took a white encased unit with a long black neck and held it in my mouth just short of the tooth being filled. After several minutes he withdrew the devise and said I was all finished. I asked, "Did that little machine utilize light to 'cure' the filling material?" "Yes, it did," he replied, and then almost defensively "but it uses harmless full spectrum light. At first we used only ultraviolet light but we found that it would interact with the photosensitive material in the filling only to a certain thickness. Full spectrum light penetrates more deeply and cures the material faster." "I was about to tell you about such a procedure mentioned in Liberman's book," I interjected, "and here I am experiencing its use!"

On March 8, 1999 I happened upon a Television News story about photodynamic therapy for lung cancer. A man's lung and all cancer that could be seen were removed surgically. The day before surgery a special drug was injected which concentrated itself in all the cancer cells. After surgery a laser light was focused from outside the body on the lung cavity – the light was drawn to all the remaining cells which had ingested the drug and the cells were destroyed. The man shown on television had been given six months to live. After above surgery, and one year later he is cancer free! Very Interesting!

There is one final note with regard to Liberman's ideas on simply being present to life, the noticer rather than the thinker of our thoughts. His concept of the Divine, of God, seems to be that God is in all that exists, and all that exists, taken collectively, *is God.* This is not a new view but a very old and classic view called Pantheism: God is All, and All is God.

Judaism, Christianity, and Islam, all conceive of God as a transcendent being, who is the creator of all that is. Judaism and Christianity teach that God is in all things as both their creator and the one who sustains them in existence. In addition, Christianity teaches that if we are open to God's will and responsive to him, he sends the Holy Spirit to dwell within us as our counselor with all his gifts. He becomes the former and informer of our inner light that shapes our perception and meaning of the outer light of the world around us.

But all things are *not* God. He is separate from his creation that has its own mode of existence, though, as we noted above, he is intimately involved in the work of his hands. He is *The Light,* the overall great healer of our entire being, the medicine of the now, and of the future!

The Medicine of Light

What I Learned and Self Help Questions for Part One

1. List three things you learned from reading or listening to The Medicine of Light that help you understand the Mind-Body-Spirit Connection in your own life experience.

2. How does each of the three things you listed in number one help you live a healthier physical, psychological, and spiritual life?

PART TWO: CONVERSATION ON ROYAL RIFE RAY TUBE, JUNE 6, 2012, DAVID TUMEY AND BERNARD FLEURY.
UPDATES BY DAVID TUMEY AS OF JULY 21, 2013

B: When I last spoke to you in 2011 on developments on the Royal Rife Ray Tube, in my 2009 edition of *Called into Life by the Light,* you indicated to me that two centers, one in Texas and one in Mexico were continually adding to Rife's original list of fifteen MORs and the viruses that they had devitalized and repeating the laboratory studies of Dr. Stafford and others. Would you please update me on the progress as of 2012? I think it was an e-mail I sent you. I am particularly interested in whether they have added two cancers B-Cell Lymphoma non-Hodgkin's and Pancreatic. A dear friend of mine has the B-Cell Lymphoma and my wife has a spot on her pancreas that has been described by two specialists, one renowned, as (1) a cyst, (2) an enlarged duct, and (3) a lesion. Both say, and we saw the film, that whatever it is it is non-cancerous but another specialized MRI is to be done on July 11th focused on the duct's description. (This test proved that there are multiple small cystic lesions seen throughout the pancreas, most or all of which appear to connect to pancreatic ducts suggesting ductal ectasia [a widening or distention of the ducts] and consistent with IMPN [Intrabilliary Mucin Producing Neoplasia]. No pancreatic ductal dilation is identified. No discrete pancreatic mass is otherwise identified. None of these areas appear to enhance significantly. No significant change in the appearance of the pancreas. Mildly dilated biliary tree probably unchanged and likely related to increased capacitance related to age and post-cholecystectomy state. No findings of clear concern). No cancer! In addition, with your permission, I will use this conversation and updates as Part Two of e-book number two of the *Called into Life by the Light* series of e-books and audio books.

D: The other thing you touched on (I assume in your e-mail) you referred to as the MORs the acronym for (Mortal

Oscillatory Rates). The "s" is a plural meaning that there are many Mortal Oscillatory Rates for the various conditions that Rife was treating. The other thing that you mentioned here, which I wanted to try to clarify, you talked about his microscope and how he watched the viruses and they would, in fact, have colors associated with them but the color of the ray machine unless I am mistaken, was always sort of a purple-blue color and that he would dial the MOR (using a frequency generator with an analog adjustment control) in order to identify the key frequency for the organism to be destroyed. So he used the colors to view the microorganism. If I recall what he was saying is, "With the light microscope you can't see viruses, you can't see small things with a light microscope because of the limitations of the wave length (of the source light). What he was able to do was using an optical heterodyning technique and ultraviolet radiation, he caused these viruses to auto-fluoresce and they were producing the light that could then be seen emanating from the organism through his instrument.

B: So in terms of what the machine itself used, it's not a question of the Rate of the MOR.

D: Right, so when I was reading a little more in your book on the medicine of light, something I never thought of before – the pathological organisms have their own light frequencies themselves and they generate the different colors, I think, as part of this autofluorescence thing. Rife had these prisms that I think are called Risley Prisms. He would turn them and that caused the light to somehow heterodyne. And when you get this organism to autofluoresce, it allows you to image something that is smaller than the normal wavelength limit – and the next step was he would use his device which produced, as I say, a sort of a violet colored purple bluish light and as I recall the earliest tubes were made from repurposed x-ray tubes with some kind of noble gas, we think it was mostly helium (possibly Argon) and they were powered by radio frequency plasma. And what he did was he turned the radio frequency plasma on and off, switching it on and off at what was referred to as the Mortal Oscillatory Rate. So he had a machine that once he was imaging, he was imaging his micro-organisms. Looking at them through the microscopes he could see them. They might be radiating, a red color, for example, then he would expose them to the ray tube. Then he would move a dial on the frequency generator and when he found the frequency that caused them to devitalize and, I think the word he used was "devitalize," he would look at the frequency and record that frequency as the MOR for that particular organism. Now there's been a lot of speculation about these numbers and of course people have changed what he referred to as the "Original" MOR frequencies. You can find them on the internet. There are hundreds of frequencies for this and that and the other, and people have referred to them as Rife's. A lot of that is kind of made up. But what we do know for a fact is that he was working with Dr. Stafford in Dayton, Ohio. Dr. Stafford (a meticulous scientist) repeated his experiments. He had the help of an engineer named Harold Leland. Harold obtained from Rife the exact frequencies he was using. I have the original resonators that Rife had given Leland, or Leland had acquired, so I know what the original frequencies really were. I've actually got the resonators. I got them from Harold. He gave them to me one day. I met with him (Leland) and Dr. Stafford back in the late 1990's. "I have no use for these Dave, and I know you are interested in them so I'm going to give you the set." I said "that's great." So I have those. I even have an original Rife X-ray Tube. It's not functional. (David had told me that the device he and Sheline had recreated was stolen – one of the devices we built (Mexican) was stolen).

B: What was it that was stolen Dave?

D: That was a device we had developed to do this sort of scanning where we would connect a subject to the device to measure biological signals while being exposed to the Rife "energy" as the computer-controlled frequency synthesizer scanned across a band of frequencies. It was based on the work of another gentleman, Dr. Lou Lala of Dayton, Ohio. We called it the "Lala" Method. Lou was a chiropractor. He was measuring, using a Pico amp meter measuring currents flowing from what we call dermatomes along the spine. He would expose the subject to the various frequencies (through a Rife machine and tube), then he would sweep across a range of frequencies, looking for spikes in his tracings. It took him hours and hours because he had to do it manually.

B: What would the spikes be associated with, David?

D: We don't know exactly what they represent other than it's a physiological response to particular frequencies. So when you're exposing the body to particular frequencies, for some reason the body responds. This is what was being tested in Hermosillo, Mexico. If a clinician were to feed these frequencies back to you, once they have identified and saved the frequencies where we see those spikes many subjects exhibited positive clinical benefit, we were also looking for dips in the signal which appeared to indicate the body was absorbing the energy at those frequencies.

B: There were certain frequencies that did certain things?

D: Each patient had a unique set of frequencies. Oftentimes there were some common frequencies in patients that represented some solid evidence of the existence of the MORs that Rife himself had identified. I don't remember them exactly (for example, a subject with a known Carcinoma might show a peak at the exact MOR Rife had himself determined was associated with that type of Carcinoma). The machine that would do this was quite complicated and involved the computer and a radio frequencies transmitter and an RF Plasma light tube system. It got out that the Doctor – we were working with an M.D., Dr. Romero – had this technology and at some point, thieves broke into his clinic and stole the equipment. Unfortunately to an untrained individual the device would be useless ad was likely scrapped or sold for parts.

B: Wow!

D: So that was a bummer! There was a second unit. We built two units (as of today 7/21/13 the second unit is in storage and not being used – a third improved device is under development).

B: I think that the second was the one you worked on – trying to get the right MOR quicker. I honestly thought it was about twenty minutes or something.

D: You know how Rife did it?

B: Trial and error?

D: Yes. Rife used a microscope and would identify the organisms he was interested in. He would then tune his frequency generator around until he found the MOR that devitalized the organism and that took a long time. So, Lou Lala wanted to speed that process up. Lou believed, in his line of thought, "Why can't I use these Pico currents which I have used before in my practice as a chiropractor, and we will broadcast the right frequencies through the body and the response from the body should indicate the correct frequency?" Rife's technique really would be in vitro where as Lou's would be in the body (in vivo). What Lou was saying is that he thought it would be more effective as Lou did it, to treat the body directly and make these measurements without having to extract, isolate, culture or study the causative agents. Lou's problem was in how he did it. He had a video camera that would monitor the output of his Pico amp meters. Then he had to turn the dials slowly like this (I believe I visually demonstrated the motion of twisting a knob with my hand). It took three hours – three or four hours. The patient would normally be sleeping and he (Dr. Lala) would be sitting there and turning the dials. So, Lou didn't have the ability to automate the process. He wasn't very technically inclined. He didn't have the ability to develop an automatic system – so we worked with Lou to assist in the development of an automated device (I believe he had the "second" device or a prototype device up to his death). We just wanted to advance

77

and simplify the process by automating it. The question was could we automate the process rather than just having a computer sitting there recording measurements that had to be taken by hand over a period of several hours?   So, one thing that I wanted to share with you, that I can provide for you, which I think that you'll find interesting. Dr. Stafford died two or three years ago.   But the year before he died, he was cleaning out a closet under his stairs, and this is right around Christmas time – I was still in San Antonio at the time so I'm going to say it had to be before 2004. He came across a box that was full of quarter inch reel to reel tapes – and apparently he didn't know what it was – he played some – and apparently he had had a tape recorder exchange with Dr. Rife and so he called up my friend, the Air Force Colonel, who was flabbergasted. Stafford immediately recovered the tapes and sent them to Colonel Heft who subsequently brought them to a laboratory and had them restored and burned onto CD's and he labeled the set *Royal Rife Speaks Again in the Year 2000.*

B: Wow!

D: And I've got these. It's kind of amazing to hear Dr. Rife's strong aggressive voice, "This is Royal Raymond Rife." I think it's the only existing recordings of Rife himself. I've got these – fifteen CD's. If you remind me – by mail I'll send you my set – I'd like to get them back when you are finished. You can listen to these tapes; hear Rife himself telling you what he was doing. One of the things you need to do if you are going to do anything with Royal Rife's technologies is that you make sure to go back to what Rife was actually doing vs. what the internet is saying. Yeah, it's crazy to hear what people are saying with respect to what Rife supposedly did, versus what he really did – very different things. Some accounts you read on line are correct and they're accurate – others are fantastic and they're just made up!

B: Just to get attention.

D: Yeah – someone's selling a machine – "works just like the Rife machine – it involves using these "foot plates". Wait a minute now, the original Rife Technology did not involve the use of "foot plates". It involved the use of a radio frequency plasma, frequency generators and RF amplifiers. Rife was a scientist and he was very meticulous in his work. He'd done a lot of things that were really new at the time. There are a handful of people who have really done a good job at recreating his equipment. Don't know much about the clinical side of this because I'm not involved clinically. I have only been involved in the engineering of it. IMPORTANT NOTE: I have never offered a device for sale to a "patient". My involvement has been developing electronic hardware on a contract engineering basis. I have never made any claims about the device being intended to diagnose, treat, cure, or prevent any disease or illness.

B: Okay

D: The design etc. Really they brought me in for my expertise in radio frequency design and in particular the generation of radio frequency plasmas.

B: I remember your mother telling me you were involved in robotics like having a man with paralysis send signals from his brain to his fingers.

D: We were using brain waves to control functional electric stimulation, so we would have devices which would cause your muscles to contract electrically and it could be controlled by brainwaves.

B: There are two places, David, that are working on a list of cancers that can be devitalized.

D: At this point I'm not aware of any continuing work. So, one of the scanning Rife machines was stolen and that clinic can no longer continue its research. I would say the machine

79

was stolen about two years ago – that would be in 2010 – and I'm not sure what the other site was or is doing (I have confirmed that this second unit is inactive and in storage as of 7/21/13). And as a matter of fact I might get part of the machine back from them to rebuild.

B: Where is the other site?

D: I don't know exactly where it was.

B: I heard of Texas.

D: I don't recall there being a site unit in Texas. I was in Texas at the time. NOTE: I believe now that the "second" device was with Dr. Lala in Ohio until his death after which it was put into storage.

B: Alright – maybe that's why I thought one of the sites was there.

D: You refer to Ohio – I think you're referring to Lou Lala – was working with his own equipment. Once we had two machines which were working. Lou had one of the working machines but I'm not sure of that because Lou was in his eighties or late seventies when I started working with him and I understand he had developed a very severe case of shingles. He continued with it for several years – I'm not sure he is alive (I confirmed he did die). I lost touch with him. I was working through my friend, the Air Force Colonel. The second machine went to Mexico which is the machine that was stolen. There was another research unit that was out in Colorado with Dr. Clifford, a microbiologist (I have this device in my possession now – it will be used in building the 2nd generation machines). He was studying the effects of the machine – how much power does it take to kill these organisms. What he did is: we built him a special unit which allowed him to dial up how much power he wanted like from one or two watts up to one hundred fifty watts of radio frequency power – very accurate – precise control – probably the nicest (research grade) machine I ever built. He called me and said, "You guys wiped out all my stock of samples" – he had all these different samples in his laboratory refrigerator. He had to replenish his entire stock due to losses that he attributed to the "Rife effect".

B: Is that what you were trying to tell me when we talked earlier up at the lake about the codes?

D: That's the Sheline experiment we did in Springfield, Ohio. That unit which was Dr. Clifford's in Colorado – I have that back. He concluded his work. He was working to determine how much power it takes to kill the organisms (BTW. Dr. Clifford concluded that as long as there is enough power to cause the tube to "light", the organisms would be destroyed – he believed the light energy was the key). The idea was to expose them to various radio frequency energy using this protocol he developed which was independently tested – by a doctor who only spoke Spanish (possibly R. Romero). I did get reports from him and he also had a gentleman in Australia who commissioned a scanning unit to be built (NOTE: Not sure this was a scanning unit, probably a standard Rife instrument) and this was just a part of the Rife technology. He sent me a series of photographs of his work). The photographs were of an external lesion on the breast that he treated with the device we built for him. In two weeks the mass dried up and fell off. It was an external lesion the size of a Big Mac! It fell off and left a very small wound there.

B: Was this the machine you worked on with Bill Sheline?

D: Oh no! The original paper which I wrote with Bill Sheline was just a reproduction of the "original" Rife Machine – so after I had a chance to meet Dr. Stafford and Harold Leland, the engineer, I set about trying to recreate a truly accurate reproduction of an original Rife Machine. I wanted to publish the paper because we wanted to make sure anyone else interested in trying to build these machines – you [can] build them yourself – could do so. We wanted to provide details in the paper describing what we did and also to give a little

81

background as to why we did it this way. We wanted to explain this is what Rife did – this is what we did and why we did this – and what Rife did was a little different than what we did. That paper was published before we built this system – around 1994. We rebuilt the unit trying to be as accurate as we could to the original – everything that Rife had. Someone who had seen the original Rife Ray Tube (Stafford and Leland) looked at it and said, "yes, this is real close to what I had back in the 1950's." That was great – it sort of put his imprimatur on it. This was exactly what we were trying to do to capture this very accurately. We even used the same vacuum tubes that he used. As I mentioned, my friend has an original Rife transmitter so he has the original equipment – bought it at an estate sale somewhere. The Transmitter is only one part of the machine. There was a presentation, around 1999 -2000 time frame, that shows you all the equipment and how that works. He uses a Rife scanning system like this – a small part of it – that's a transmitter.

B: I lost the presentation on my computer.

D: I have it with me – I'll put it back on your computer. Let me share with you something that convinces me that the Rife effect is more than just radio frequency energy – and that light actually plays a larger role. So the idea behind the radio frequency energy was to create a plasma inside this tube which is often referred to as the Helium/Argon gas – the plasma – what you are doing is exciting these electrons in the atoms of this noble gas to move to higher orbits. When those electrons return to their natural state they give off a photon of light in a particular frequency – and that's when the plasma glows. So what we did was, and this was a kind of accident – we had gotten hold of a double walled Faraday cage – six foot by four foot – pretty good size – we had used that to put a copper screen on all sides that's grounded. We had a second wall of copper screen outside the first. The idea of a Faraday screen like that will prevent electric magnetic radiation from entering. As you would expect, if you would take a transistor radio and tune to a station from inside the cage, when you close the doors, that would be it. All you'd hear was static. Because the radio waves can't penetrate the cage – they're stuck on the outside of it. As I recall Bill Sheline came across this accidentally. He wanted to write a follow-up paper but he never finished it. He died about two years ago – complications from diabetes. But this one day he had put the Rife Equipment inside the cage – same equipment we described in the paper – and he had a receiver on the outside with an antenna. Because the Rife Equipment does broadcast to some degree radio frequency signals, we could hear it on the Receiver. But what you hear on the Receiver is the MOR, so if you are using a 1000 cycles per. second MOR you're hearing a 1000 cycles per. second MOR on the Receiver because the Receiver demodulates the radio frequencies. So he said to me, "You watch this. I am going to close the doors on the cage." And when he closed both of the cages the Receivers stopped receiving the signal from the Transmitter. But when you touched the (receiver) antenna with your hand, for example, you could hear the MOR frequencies again through the receiver. So what is interesting is it didn't seem to affect the antenna if you touched it to inanimate objects like when you touched the metal – I think it was a microphone stand – you could not hear the frequencies then, but as soon as a human being touched the antenna to the body (i.e. living tissue, you could again hear the MOR frequency). It was definitely stronger in some parts of the body than others.

B: There was some energy there?

D: There was some energy there that was escaping the Faraday Cage. Now we know that light can get out of the cage because the holes in the screen are large enough. It was like a copper window screen. There certainly is an energy that is able to penetrate a Faraday Cage and a lot of people have attributed this energy to something being produced by the RF plasma in the tube. They think the discharge tube kind of acts as a negative resister and that makes a sort of strange antenna and that's really why we need the plasma. But there's more to it

83

than that. I don't know that I understand exactly what's happening there. But, I thought that that was fascinating.

B: Teilhard de Chardin says there are two forms of energy. One is psychic and the other is physical. He calls it psychic energy because it doesn't occupy space or have weight but it is a power that causes things to happen. There is power there. What you were perceiving outside the cage, he says, was the ultimate energy, psychic energy. It glows. It is light in its most basic form – psychic energy. As you go back farther and farther in evolution the particles become smaller and smaller in terms of mass or behavior until finally there is no measurement at all in terms of mass or behavior but there is something there that glows. And when you get back to where that energy is centered in one being, you've arrived at God. Some say that Faith and Reason don't go together – de Chardin says they do. They are two aspects of the same Phenomenon.

D: That is kind of interesting. I would agree that there is something. A living organism has the ability to demodulate this signal even though a Radio Receiver wasn't able to do so – something about the living organism. But, there it was, a light escaping from the box. You could see the light – that it was running. You could see the light – it was not a light that could burn your skin or tan it. I've worked around these things for a long time and I've never had any ill effects and Bill Sheline didn't either. Yes, it was an interesting experiment. At some point I need to sit down and write it up. I talked to his wife and she said it would be okay for me to credit Bill on the paper for this discovery.

B: It's great to get all these things done before things pass away – you know stuff disappears.

D: Unfortunately most of the folks who were involved in this, I'm going to say it was about 1992-93, when I first became involved, were in their 60's or 70's already. I know that Dr. Stafford is gone and Harold was older by several years so he's probably gone also.

B: Don Higby, the MD I was talking to you about, was head of Oncology and Hematology at Bay State Hospital in Springfield and a Professor at Tufts University. He saved my life several times. I went over there with things. One time I had a red line running up one leg – he sent me right over to be tested. He's retired now but has kept his license. He was fascinated with your work. He was particularly interested in finding out if there was any other list of cancers developed in addition to the ones that were mentioned in your work with Sheline at the two other places, that I mentioned to you earlier in this discussion and which you gave me an update on. It's a shame if more research is not done on enlarging the list of cancers which can be devitalized and destroyed without harming healthy tissue around the malignancy. It would benefit a whole lot of people. This lady I know is only fifty five years old and has a persistent BC non- Hodgkin's Lymphoma. She can't have any more radiation treatments without destroying her healthy body tissue in her back because the cancer is too deep and there's some of it left.

D: The only options Doctors have today (to treat degenerative illness) is you can (cut it out), burn it out with radiation or you can poison it! That's all. They completely ignore electronics – electronic therapy. When you think about it the body is an electro-chemical machine. It involves chemistry. There's no question there's a lot of chemistry going on, a lot of chemical processes. But there's also a lot of electricity in the body.

B: Well it's true that there's really nothing solid in the body. Everything is in constant motion, but the movement is so rapid that our naked eyes cannot pick it up.

D: Actually we're mostly empty space. When you split the atoms apart you get these elementary particles and exchange particles such as Gluons that represent binding energy fields. The particles keep getting smaller and smaller until you get

85

down to pure information – nothing physical. Essentially medicine has ignored the electro-chemical part of the body.

B: Why are they ignoring it? All the new diagnostic machines that work in terms of accurate diagnosis and some that are curative are all light based. The CAT Scan, MRI, and Ultra Sound, utilize light based technology. Sound waves are basically light.

D: There are a lot of diagnostic technologies which use a photon of some kind or other. I think you are seeing people looking at light as a possible source of therapy. You have light for pain. They use the light in plasmas for disinfecting rooms and things.

B: That's right David. At the hospital where my daughter is a charge nurse they have a special germ killing sanitizing machine that uses ultra violet light to sanitize rooms especially after patients who had very contagious ailments vacate them. This professor from Amherst College, Arthur Zajonc wrote a fascinating book entitled *Catching the Light* in 1993. It's a treatise on the very concept of light. Although he is a professor of physics and a specialist in quantum physics he goes much beyond what is conventionally thought of as the realm of physics. His approach to Light, I capitalize the word in my book because Light has a very special meaning to him, is much like Teilhard de Chardin's approach to ultimate reality. He is a synthesizer who has the gift of being able to bring to bear the insights of history, science, mathematics, religion, and art on the concept of light from biblical times to the modern era. As it says on the jacket of his book, "Zajonc brings together the multifaceted strands of human experience to light the way to a new understanding of ourselves and our cosmos."

David, I guess the culture today views anything spiritual as superstition and one thing I'm most impressed about Pope, John Paul II, is that in 1998 encyclicals *Fides et Ratio*, Faith and Reason, he writes that faith without reason leads to superstition and reason without faith lacks hope. Why should you do anything? Reason doesn't answer the "why".

D: Well that's right – The existence of our universe, which is vast, does not exclude the existence of a Deity. If you were to walk along the shore of an ocean and this thing washed up onto the sand, an iPhone, you would say that this thing required some form of engineering by somebody. It's too complicated to just come together. That would be like saying that the winds of a hurricane blowing through a junkyard could create the parts and assemble a 747airplane. The human body and animals in general are so much more complex than this, and yet we immediately want to assume that there was no designer, no engineering or intelligent creator. The fact is, when we look at how amazing we are, we look at ancient human fossils and then compare them to modern human bodies, we cannot deny evolution. We can't deny the fact that things will change. Biological entities will adapt to their environment. So, we've got that mechanism designed into us. But I think that evolution is just part of our design. I think that we are designed to adapt.

B: That's what de Chardin says. He defines evolution as the ascent to consciousness. We're the most recent living development on this planet.

D: I think that the whole thing was designed – in many ways. What's interesting – and many physicists will not admit this – is that the numbers work out so well. It appears that someone has set down before and figured this all out mathematically. The math does work so well describing our physical world, that it is a tool that was probably used to design the whole universe.

B: Do you think that maybe that this is why some of these light-based technologies work so well, because light is the basic stuff of the universe? They are tied in with something deeper in the universe: the way the universe is actually set up.

D: That's right. The body itself has more components to it than just chemistry. We can create. When we can create with a pharmaceutical a chemical reaction within your body, but I also think that light will do that, magnetism will do that, electricity will do that, even a radio wave frequency can be considered to be light. We think of light as a very narrow part of the electromagnetic spectrum. Light is an electro-magnetic radiation. We define light as a very narrow range, but the spectrum goes all the way from Direct Current, through radio waves, light, x-rays, gamma rays to infinity. (Using my hands to depict and point out parts of the electromagnetic spectrum) We've got your gamma rays here, your x-rays here, your microwaves, your visible rays which your eyes can receive, lower frequencies which radios can pick up and transmit, and you keep going down to the audio frequency range and you get down to zero. But, it's all electro-magnetic radiation. It all behaves the same way.

B: That's right. I have been exposed to photo therapy treatment for my eyes. Dr. Lizotte uses a Spectro-Receptivity Trainer and flashes in small ball shaped disks the entire rainbow spectrum. Then he picks out which colors you seem to need most. Believe it or not I was cross eyed. It never showed. My right eye was a lazy eye which focused with my left eye. After a series of treatments my right eye focused on its own. My peripheral vision greatly improved and my overall vision which was 20/40 came back to 20/20 normal vision. My right eye was hard wired into focusing on its own. You do need to have maintenance every three or four years to keep the optic nerves fully activated barring anything like cataracts, etc. I haven't had any treatments for more than three years. The hardwiring with regard to the right eye focusing on its own continues. But because I have not kept up my eye exercises Dr. Lizotte gave me nor had any maintenance treatments, and used my glasses most of the time, not reading without them in bright natural light, my overall acuity has diminished.

D: Oh sure. When you think of color you are dealing with the wave length of electro-magnetic radiation. The shorter the wave length and the higher the frequency, the closer you are toward the blue end, ultra violet. The longer the wave and the lower the frequency, you are at the red (infra-red) end. But if you look at it as an electro-magnetic radiation and essentially that's a transverse wave with a magnetic and electric field at 90 degrees relative to each other, you've got an electric field and a magnetic field, and as one field increases another collapses. It's self supporting. It doesn't need a medium in which to travel in order for it to propagate through the air – you don't need an ether – so what carries the wave? Michaelson put the arrow in the ether coffin. It didn't exist and Einstein proved it with his theory of special relativity. Here's an experiment you can replicate:

If you're driving in a car at fifty miles an hour and I throw a ball at you as you're going by at five miles an hour, I would measure the speed of the ball at five miles an hour relative to me but you would register the speed at fifty five miles an hour. The speed of the car, plus the speed of the ball. Does that make sense?

B: I don't get it!

D: Let's say the car is not moving. I throw the ball at you at five miles an hour. I measure the ball.

B: Are the cars side by side?
What do you think?

Conversation on Royal Rife Ray Tube, June 6, 2012, David Tumey and Bernard Fleury.
Updates by David Tumey as of July 21, 2013

What I Learned and Self Help Questions for Part Two

1. If I was suffering from a particular form of cancer, why would it be very important for my cure to have the frequency generator generate the Mortal Oscillatory Rate (MOR), the frequency that caused my cancer to "devitalize"?

2. Why is it really important to me if I hope to gain any sort of health benefit from Royal Rife's technology that I know what Rife actually did versus what the internet is saying? Listening to the fifteen CDs in "Royal Rife Speaks Again in 2000" is a start.

3. What does the light frequency which escaped the Faraday Cage and could be sensed when a person placed his/her hand on the Antenna indicate in terms of the presence of psychic energy, the form of energy that doesn't occupy space or have weight but is a power that causes things to happen?

PART THREE: DR. ROYAL RAYMOND RIFE: THE MAN, HIS MICROSCOPES, BX, THE CANCER CAUSING MICROBE, AND FREQUENCY INSTRUMENTS

Introduction

Citations Permission for quoting from *Royal R. Rife Speaks Again in the Year 2000.*

On Sunday March 24, 2013, at 11:48 a.m., David Tumey e-mailed Edward Heft, Sr. the copyright holder of the Royal Rife Speaks CD set. (Kinnerman Foundation).

"This fall, I loaned my CD of 'Royal Rife speaks' to author Bernie Fleury....he is working on a new book (and e-book) *The Medicine of Light* and would like to quote with proper citation from the 'Royal Rife Speaks' CD set. He is asking permission to do so and I told him I needed to speak to you about it..."

On Sunday March 24, 2013 at 2:59 p.m., Edward Heft , Sr. replied by e-mail: "CERTAINLY...the only desire I see is to get the truth out!!! I am glad to hear of someone doing this vital work and would support and encourage anyone who does ethical and honorable work. - Ed"

Thank you, David and Ed, for allowing me to tell Rife's story in his own words.

In my e-book number 2 – *The Mind-Body-Spirit Connection in the Medicine of Light* there are other written resources which confirm and amplify what Rife says about his life and work. It is a story that many persons, including those in the medical field, are still not aware of or are still consciously suppressing it. It is a story that needs to be told again!

"Dr. Royal Rife Speaks again in year 2000"
(Copyrighted 2002)
History of the Tapes

There had been no indications of any audio tapes ever being recorded of Dr. Rife telling about his experiences using his microscopes and Frequency Instruments – until !!!!--- Early March 2000, at 5 PM, when a telephone call was received. An excited Dr. R.P. Stafford, M.D., announced that while cleaning out a closet in his home, he discovered eight reel-to-reel audio tapes (Scotch Brand Magnetic Tape 190A[1-3" & 3 ea. 5" reels] & NO Brand name [4-5" reels]) from the Rife Labs, dated back in the late 50's. John Crane had sent the tapes to him, about the time Dr. Stafford was going to do his rat tests to evaluate the effectiveness of the Rife Frequency Instrument (RFI). Dr. Stafford, being very busy at that point of his life with his professional and civic involvement, put them into safe storage, without opening nor listening to the tapes. The reel boxes were still taped together when received from Dr. Stafford.

Reproduction Procedure: These forty-plus year old magnetic tapes were opened one at a time, and then played n a new reel-to-reel Teac Model R2000R Tape Deck. The deck was chosen for its rolling Amorphous Record and Playback Heads. The output signal was fed into a Mackie Micro-series 1402VLZ 14 channel (80hz-12Khz), outputted into a Yamaha PSR-8000 Composers workstation (32hz/12db gain to 16khz) pls Q factor 0.1 to 12/1.0 to 12 all band frequency range output back into the Mackie, inputted to Fostex D108 Hard drive Recorder and Fostex CR300 Master CD Duplicator. All this effort was required to optimize Dr. Rife's voice, while reducing the hiss and poor tonal quality –there was considerable bleed through from the reverse side track and adjoining layers of tape. John Crane had spliced sections of different brands of tapes together which, had failed due to age, and had to be reattached. Every effort was made to reproduce all the origin verbiage, including repeats, using the latest sound technology, attempting to emulate Dr. Rife's Very High

92

Standards. Premium CD's were copied on a CD3701 Media Form Standalone, Robotic Auto-CD Duplicator with copyright and watermark protection. Every hour that you hear from each CD, has 8-15 hours of sound conditioning refined by Mr. Billie Coldiron. "Thanks for a superb job, Billie."

Citations For Royal Rife Timeline

Power Pedia – PESWIKIA was created July 22, 2011. The Power Pedia is a power encyclopedia or set of pages of informative articles arranged to provide you information on various energy – a free-for-all community-built Free Energy's power encyclopedia Power Pedia.

All content is available under GNU Free Documentation License 1.6. Retrieved from http://peswiki.com/index.php/PowerPedia:Royal_Raymond_Ri fe.

When I entered this link on October 7, 2014 the following message appeared: "There is currently no text on this page. You can search for this page title in other pages or edit this page." "Search for this title" yielded "There is no page titled 'Power Pedia: Royal_ Raymond Rife." "you can create this page." When I clicked on that I saw, "The action you have requested is limited to users in the groups user."

I had printed the Timeline in the summer of 2014 so I had it to use as I cite below.

I am fully aware that information that readers can add to or subtract from cannot be used as the sole source of anything. However, I have utilized the content of the Biographical Timeline of Royal R. Rife's life compiled by A. Walter in May 1998 as a baseline that the following sources also cite, agree with, and or amplify. In addition to A. Walter's Timeline my primary quoted sources are:

1. "A New Light on Cancer": Sub-Title in Part One: "The Medicine of Light" in this e-book.

2. Bernard J. Fleury and David Tumey Conversation on Royal Rife Ray Tube, June 6, 2012.

3. "Dr. Royal R. Rife Speaks Again in the Year 2000."

4. The Annual Report of the Board of Regents of the Smithsonian Institution for 1944.

I use the following three sources as "also cite" what A. Walter does and my primary four quoted sources do. I purchased both of Barry Lynes cited books.

1. *Rife's World of Electromedicine*, by Barry Lynes 2009.

2. *Royal Raymond Rife Discovers Cancer Cure* – an article by Jeff Rense.

3. *The Cancer Cure That Worked*, by Barry Lynes (Thirteenth printing, May 2011).

The Timeline of Royal R. Rife's Life and Accomplishments A. Walker (5/98)

Enhanced and Amended by Bernard J. Fleury (10/14)

Rife was born in Elkhorn, Nebraska, and in 1913 married and moved to San Diego, where he was employed as a family chauffeur. He is reported to have worked for one of the German optical companies (Zeiss or Leitz) for a few years before World War One, and to have served in the US Navy during this war.

Timeline

[Note from A. Walter: He discovered an effective cure for cancer and many other diseases. Was he the greatest hero of the century? Read on and see what happened.]

1888   Born in Elkhorn, Nebraska.

1913   Married. Moves to San Diego. A man of varied interests: ballistics, racing auto constructions, optics and microscopy.

1915-1918   Serves in the Navy. Sent to investigate foreign laboratories by the United States Government.

1920   Begins to investigate the possibilities of electric treatment of diseases. Timken, owner of Timken Roller Bearing Company, and Bridges of Bridges Carriage Company, provide funds to establish a laboratory and to finance his research. Begins research on tuberculosis.

1922   Begins cancer research.

1929   October. Stock market crash. Two weeks later, Nov. 3, 1929, the San Diego Union carries an article announcing that Rife has built a microscope capable of staining living viruses with light to make them visible! (Today this is called bioluminescence.)

1931   Two men join Rife in his work: Dr. Arthur 1. Kendall, Director of Medical Research at Northwestern University and Dr. Milbank Johnson of Pasadena Hospital. Dr. Alvin G. Frood, President of the American Association of Pathologists also becomes active in Rife's research.

1931 Nov.22   L.A. Times announces the discovery of a "filterable typhoid bacillus" being

95

light-stained and observed to "change back into non-filterable form", as seen through a powerful new microscope developed by Royal Raymond Rife that could directly observe living bacterium and viruses.

1932 May 3-4   Kendall speaks before the Association of American Physicians at Johns Hopkins University telling of the preliminary successes with Rife's methods and treatments. Dr. Thomas Rivers, virologist and bacteriologist, Director of the Rockefeller Institute – a primary source of funding for medical research -- and Dr. Hans Zinsser, call Kendall a liar to his face in front of the assembled crowd. They couldn't replicate Rife's discoveries with River's microscope due to its much lower magnification and the fact that the electron microscope killed live bacteria and viruses. Rivers simply could not physically see what Rife could with his new microscope and its ability to stain living viruses with light. Rivers never known to have used Rife's method or instruments.

1932 July 5-7   Dr. Edward C. Rosenow of the Mayo Clinic's Division of Experimental Bacteriology witnesses Rife's results and becomes a supporter. But, after Rife's trial Rosenow will leave Rife sometime after 1994. Cf. 1939 June 12 entry and 1944 Smithsonian Report Acknowledgment of Dr. Edward C. Rosenow as one of the contributors to Rife's report. As a filtrationist (one who believes in pleomorphism) Rosenow was a maverick among biologists up to his death at ninety four in the 1960s.

1932 Nov. 30   Rife isolates the filtrable virus of carcinoma. "Angle of refraction (polarization) 123/16 degrees; length 1/15 micron; breadth 1/20 micron, color by chemical refraction red-purple." Pleomorphism also established.

1932   By end of the year "Rife can destroy the typhus bacteria, the polio virus, the herpes virus, the cancer virus and other viruses in culture and in experimental animals."

1933   Rife completes the "universal microscope." A resolution of 31,000 times and a magnification of 60,000 times – first produced in 1932.

The War Between Monomorphism and Pleomorphism which began in 1932 continues. Monomorphism (noun) means of the same or of an essentially similar type of structure. Pleomorphic (adjective) means the occurrence of two or more forms in the life cycle of an organism. The definitions are from Webster's College Dictionary, 2000. Rife proved that Pleomorphism (the so called filterable forms) exist and are the causative factor of cancers and some other diseases listed in the 1944 Smithsonian Report under the section entitled, *The Universal Microscope,* pages 207-216. Pages 208-209 and 214-216 are included in this e-book. Pages 209-213 go into detail about the mechanics of the Universal Microscope, how earlier Rife microscopes worked and what was discovered by them like the presence of the filter passing forms of Bacillus Typhosus. These five pages also compare and contrast what "ordinary microscopes" could reveal compared to what Rife's microscopes, especially the Universal Microscope could reveal. Details of the Universal Microscope are presented in pages 208-213, and 214-216.

1933 July   Dr. Karl Meyer, Director of the Hooper Foundation for Medical Research of UCSF joins Rife's team.

97

1934 Summer   The first cancer clinic using Rife technology. A special University of Southern California Medical Research Committee chaired by Milbank Johnson is formed to oversee the research. Committee members are: Whalen Morrison, Chief Surgeon of the Santa Fe Railway. George C. Dock, M.D. George C. Fischer, M.D., Children's Hospital of New York, Arthur 1. Kendall, Dr. Zite, M.D., professor of pathology of Chicago University. Rufus B. Yon Klein Schmidt, President of USC [University of Southern California].

Also in attendance:

Dr. James Couche of San Diego.

Dr. Carl Meyer, Ph.D. of the Hooper Foundation, SF.

Dr. Kopps of the Metabolic Clinic in La Jolla.

The clinic is held at the Scripps Institute in La Jolla, California. Sixteen terminally ill people are treated. Fourteen are cured: in three months, the other two are cured in six months. Did the cancer cures last?

Later Rife was to prove that the cancer microbe had four forms BX (carcinoma), BY(sarcoma). Monococcoid, and crytomyces Pleomorphis fungi. Rife who had proven pleomorphism over and over again reiterated that any of the three forms can be changed back to the BX within a day and a half period. (See *Rife Speaks in 2000* CDs, numbers 4, 10, 13 and in Part One of this e-book, Topic number 16, "A New Light on Cancer").

What was learned at the 1934 Summer Clinic?

(*Rife Speaks in 2000* CDs, Smithsonian Report of 1944,and Rife's 1953 Report, all of which were my sources, and sources of Lynes' citations in *The Cancer Cure That Worked,* pages 60-61, and 64-65.

1. The Summer 1934 Treatments
    --Exposed to frequency for three minutes every third day. Time schedule needed to assure that toxins from dead cancer micro-organisms could be absorbed or cast off by person's lymphatic system.
    --Treatment harmless to noncancerous tissue and painless.
    --Frequency instrument set at the correct MOR (Mortal Oscillatory Rate) for BX. The correct frequency of light was the same color as the cancer BX virus. The matching of colors absolutely necessary if the cancer microorganism was to be devitalized (destroyed),

2. The lack of support personnel (nurses and secretaries) meant that records kept were not complete enough to attract non-attending and disbelieving fellow Doctors and Scientists. Milbank Johnson, himself, attested to this fact.
    --Clinic was a first step. Cancers were cured. But frequency instrument (especially the ease of arriving at the correct MOR had to be improved time-wise and stability-wise.
    --Replication by other scientist willing to correctly use Rife's Microscope and Frequency Instrument was justified and needed.

Detection of Mortal Oscillatory Rates (MORs) In Vivo by David Tumey, Engineer

After Rife perfected his light-heterodyning technique for imaging live bacteria and viruses microscopically, he next discovered that a radio frequency (RF) plasma (light) could

99

destroy the pathogens if it was modulated at a resonant frequency. This frequency he called the Mortal Oscillatory Rate or MOR. To discover frequencies that had the desired destructive effect on a given targeted pathogen, he would observe the bug under his microscope while he painstakingly tuned a frequency generator until devitalization was observed. He would then repeat these experiments until a precise MOR could be determined. These were the treatment frequencies he used as part of his therapy. He developed his cancer-fighting protocols through this technique having discovered that certain forms of cancer could be transmitted via a filterable virus – a virus that could be destroyed in vivo if a patient was exposed to this properly modulated RF plasma energy field.

The question of course is: *Is there a more efficient way to obtain the MOR frequencies, and further, can the MOR frequencies be obtained in vivo?*

In the late 90's, early 2000's Dr. Lu Lala of Dayton, Ohio began work trying to solve this problem. Dr. Lu is a Chiropractor and had been practicing medicine for his entire adult life. He used to work with instruments called galvanometers and Pico ammeters used in measuring small electrical potentials and currents. As a Chiropractor, he used these devices to diagnose subluxations (pinched nerves). His idea was to locate electrical sensors along spinal dermatomes connected to a multi-channel Pico amp meter. His protocol called for tuning a frequency generator across a band of potential MORs while observing the electrical activity of the selected dermatomes. He would mark any resonant frequencies that were acquired as potential therapeutic frequencies. Thus his idea was to "Scan" a human subject and determine in vivo all of the various resonant MORs that would subsequently be used in later treatments. To help automate his procedure, he used a video camera with time-lapse photography and a programmable frequency generator. He would run a scan on a patient (which normally would take about two hours) then review the video that showed both the MOR frequency and dermatome response. He would record

100

the actual frequencies of interest in a lab notebook. This review process took several hours to complete and was done after a scan had been recorded.

When I got involved in the project around 2001/02 timeframe, I developed a software algorithm that completely automated the entire process. Using a computer, and a computer-controlled frequency generator, my system would scan a patient and automatically record the electrical response from the Pico amp meter. Once the scan was complete, all the relevant data was already in the computer, all the operator had to do was to go through the data and "click" on the potential MOR frequencies which were subsequently loaded into a therapy table that would be used in future treatments. This technique reduced the entire scan, recording and analysis time to approximately one hour. Since this time, I have developed an improved system that is anticipated to reduce these times to about 20 minutes.

Currently (2012), there are two working prototypes. One is located in a medical clinic in Hermosillo, Mexico and is being operated by a Dr. Romero. The other is located in a lab in Dayton, Ohio where research into this technique continues.

1935   Rife builds a smaller microscope that can be mass produced.

May - June: Dr. O. Cameron Gruner of Montreal replicates Rife & Kendall's cancer   pleomorphism.

June: Four insurance companies are interested in financing Rife provided the   International   Cancer Foundation gave its approval. Dr. Mildred Schram, Secretary of the. Foundation, after visiting Rife's lab, stipulates conditions for acceptance which have nothing to do with Rife's work. Rife doesn't have time to be sidetracked. Result: the Cancer Foundation never funds any of Rife's work.

September: A new version of the Rife Frequency Ray is completed. October: Drs. Walker & Meyer of The Hooper Clinic, SF, using Rife's microscope and "Beam Ray" replicate his cures.

Rife had begun using his initial Frequency Instrument on animals in 1932 as in the citation insert immediately after the 1959-60 Timeline entry. Rife had begun to use the Frequency Instrument on humans for the first time at the 1934 clinic. The new Frequency Instrument used some parts from the previous one.

After the completion of the 1935 Instrument, it had to have its MOR calibrations synchronized with the previous version.

Also Rife wanted better control (stability) of a selected frequency and variable control of it so that it was quicker and easier to match the vibratory rate of the Frequency Instrument frequency, with the rate of the pathogenic organism (like BX) that Rife wanted to devitalize (destroy).

Rife describes in CD number four of *Rife Speaks in 2000* precisely much of which he later incorporated in his 1953 Report.

My prescription way back in 1921-22, when I first started to work on this, that when the causative agent of this malignancy (cancer) was found it would be found to be caused by a microorganism, and, not unlikely, that micro- organism, a so called non-pathogenic, we have with us at all times, that the shift in the metabolism in the individual would alter that organism into something else. That I proved definitely years later. So I developed the First Microscope for that work, studying those tissues....
The Frequency Instrument has more penetration than x-ray....

Every virus organism requires a different frequency according to its own constituents, its' primordial cell or predominant chemical factor. You see, practically all of these viruses are made up of what we call a predominant chemical factor and all have radicals, (that is) certain percentages of radical particles that are in them. We disregard those because the predominant chemical factor is the one that carries. Like I say, I believe sincerely and honestly, that it is the chemical constituents of this particular virus, or primordial cell as we term it, of the pathogenic bacteria that are enacting upon the unbalanced cell metabolism of the human body that in actuality produce the disease....

The effect of a disease on an individual depends greatly upon the balance of the metabolism of that individual from a neutral PH. Because I sincerely believe if the body is (perfectly balanced or poised), an absolute normal PH, it is susceptible to no diseases. Because our test tubes show that they won't let anything grow with a normal PH.

[Author's note: Webster's College Dictionary defines PH as "the symbol for the logarithm of the reciprocal of hydrogen ion concentration in gram atoms per liter, used to describe the acidity or alkalinity of a chemical (solution on a scale of 0 (more acidic) to 14 (more alkaline)."]

Levels of acidity play an important role in our digestive system and in our overall bodily well being as well as in our agricultural practices.

November: Dr. Johnson opens a second clinic to test cures with the same incredible results as the first clinic.

1936   June 2: William Donner, President of the International Cancer Research Institute turns down Johnson's application for research funds.

1937   July: Rife moves into his new lab on Alcott St. in Point Lorna, built for him by his sponsor, Henry Timkin.

1937   September - May: Johnson's third clinic resulting in the same, identical cures. There is mounting pressure to go public. But Rife and his academic advisors, being cautious and recognizing the inevitable resistance from medical orthodoxy, are determined to gather as much irrefutable and massive statistical evidence as possible.

1937   Drs. Couche of San Diego, Gruner of Montreal are using Rife's Beam Ray with great success. In the fall Rife hires an engineer, Phil Hoyland, to help start a company for manufacturing the Beam Ray.

1938   The Rife Beam Ray Co. is in operation. Fourteen machines are built. Two go to England, one goes to Dr. Richard Hamer of the Paradise Valley Sanitarium, one to Dr. Arthur Yale, two to Arizona doctors, and eight to Southern California doctors. Dr. Hammer cures an eighty-two year old from Chicago of terminal cancer. Through this man, Morris Fishbein, head of the American Medical Association in Chicago learns of Rife and his work. Fishbein visits Rife. Wants to buy in. Rife and his associates turn him down. [This creates Fishbein's prime revenge motivation for targeting Rife for indictment and the ultimate destruction of his work].

1938   The J.C Burnett Laboratory in New Jersey, which had done research on electronic energy medicine and its curative effects on the human body, is burnt to the ground. Burnett's wife is a member of the Timken family, which had originally financed Royal Rife. The lab is burned while Burnett and his wife are visiting Rife!

     The American Medical Association indicts Rife for fraudulent medical practices.

1939   June 12: Opening day of Rife's trial.   During his testimony, Rife is so nervous he cannot stop shaking. A doctor recommends he take a drink to calm himself. Rife's alcoholism begins and hounds him for the rest of his life.

During the trial and afterwards the American Medical Association visits all doctors involved with Rife. "Those who didn't stop using the Frequency Instruments lose their medical license. Dr. Hamer quickly returns his instrument. Dr. Gruner returns his. Dr. Couche defies the American Medical Association into the 1950's and his membership and his license are revoked. Many other doctors associated with Rife turn their backs on him including Drs. Drood, Rosenow, & Meyer. Rife nevertheless wins the case. The American Medical Association pays off Kendall in Baltimore "about" $200,000.   He goes to Mexico, loses his property there, comes back to the United States to live in La Jolla, California and in 1940 Kendall dies.

1944   Milbank Johnson dies under suspicious circumstances. Two federal inspectors conclude in the 1950's to 60's era, that he was likely poisoned. Reputedly, as head of his academic committee, he was to present the long delayed Rife findings to the American Medical Association the following day. All Rife's records kept by his academic committee are destroyed. The committee disbands.

ANNUAL REPORT OF THE
BOARD OF REGENTS OF

THE SMITHSONIAN
INSTITUTION

1944

The Universal Microscope (Pages 207-208)

It is not only a reasonable supposition , but already, in one instance, a very successful and highly commendable achievement on the part of Dr. Royal Raymond Rife of San Diego, California, who, for many years, has built and worked with light microscopes which far surpass the theoretical limitations of the ordinary variety of instrument, all the Rife scopes possessing superior ability to attain high magnification with accompanying high resolution. The largest and most powerful of these, the universal microscope, developed in 1933, consists of 6,682 parts and is so called because of its adaptability in all fields of microscopical work, being fully equipped with separate substage condenser units for transmitted and monochromatic beam, dark-field, polarized and slit-ultra illumination, including also a special device for crystallography. The entire optical system of lenses and prisms as well as the illuminating units are made of block-crystal quartz, quartz being especially transparent to ultraviolet radiations.

The illuminating unit used for examining the filterable forms of disease organisms contains fourteen lenses and prisms, three of which are in the high-intensity incandescent lamp, four in the Risley prism, and seven in the achromatic condenser which incidentally, has a numerical aperture of 1.40. Between the source of light and the specimen are subtended two circular, wedge-shaped, block-crystal quartz prisms for the purpose of polarizing the light passing through the specimen, polarization being the practical application of the theory that light waves vibrate in all planes perpendicular to the direction in which they are propagated. Therefore, when light comes into contact with a polarizing prism, it is divided or split into two beams, one of which is refracted to such an extent that it is reflected to the side of the prism without, of course, passing through the prism while the second ray, bent considerably less, is thus enabled to pass through the prism to illuminate the

106

specimen.   When the quartz prisms on the universal microscope, which may be rotated with vernier control through 360 degrees, are rotated in opposite directions, they serve to bend the transmitted beams of light at variable angles of incidence while, at the same time, a spectrum is projected up into the axis of the microscope, or rather a small portion of a spectrum since only a part of a band of color is visible at any one time.   However, it is possible to proceed in this way from one end of the spectrum to the other, going all the way from the infrared to the ultraviolet.   Now, when that portion of the spectrum is reached in which both the organism and the color band vibrate in exact accord, one with the other, a definite characteristic spectrum is emitted by the organism.   In the case of the filter-passing form of the *Bacillus typhosus,* for instance, a blue spectrum is emitted and the plane of polarization deviated plus 4.8 degrees.   The predominating chemical constituents of the organism are next ascertained after which the quarts prisms are adjusted or set, by means of vernier control, to minus 4.8 degrees (again in the case of the filter-passing form of the *Bacillus typhosus*) so that the opposite angle of refraction may be obtained.   A monochromatic beam of light, corresponding exactly to the frequency of the organism (for Dr. Rife has found that each disease organism responds to and has a definite and distinct wave length, a fact confirmed by British medical research workers) is then sent up through the specimen and the direct transmitted light, thus enabling the observer to view the organism stained in its true chemical color and revealing its own individual structure in a field which is brilliant with light.

The B. X. Virus (Pages 214-216)

The discovery of the B.X. Virus involved more than 20,000 laboratory cultures of carcinoma which were grown and studied over a period of seven years by Dr. Rife and his assistants in what, at the time, appeared to be a fruitless effort to isolate the filter-passing form, or virus, which Dr. Rife believed to be present in this condition.   Then, in 1932, the reactions in growth of bacterial cultures to light from the rare gasses were observed, indicating a new approach to the problem. Accordingly, blocks of tissue one-half centimeters square, taken from an unulcerated breast carcinoma, were placed in triple-sterilized **K** Medium and these cultures incubated at 37 degrees **C**. When no results were forthcoming, the culture tubes were placed in a circular loop filled with argon gas to a pressure of 14 millimeters, and a current of 5,000 volts applied for 24 hours, after which the tubes were placed in a two inch water vacuum and incubated at 37 degrees **C**. for 24 hours. Using a specially designed 1.12 dry lens, equal in amplitude of magnification to the 2-mm. apochromatic oil-immersion lens, the cultures were then examined under the universal microscope, at a magnification of 10,000diameters, where very much animated, purplish-red, filterable forms, measuring less than one-twentieth of a micron in dimension, were observed. Carried through fourteen transplants from **K** Medium to **K** Medium, this **B. X.** virus remained constant; inoculated into 426 Albino rats, tumors "with all the true pathology of neoplastic tissue" were developed. Experiments conducted in the Rife Laboratories have established the fact that these characteristic diplococci are found in the blood monocytes in 92 percent of all cases of neoplastic diseases. It has also been demonstrated That the virus of cancer, like the viruses of other diseases, can be easily changed from one form to another by means of altering the media upon which it is grown. With the first change in media, the **B. X.** virus becomes considerably enlarged although its purplish-red color remains unchanged. Observation of the organism with an ordinary microscope is made possible bay a second alteration of the media. A third change is undergone upon asparagus base media where the **B. X.** virus is transformed from its filterable state into cryptomyces pleomorphia fungi, these fungi being identical morphologically both macroscopically and microscopically to that of the orchid and of the mushroom. And yet a fourth change may be said to take place when this cyrptomyces pleomorphia, permitted to stand as a stock culture for the period of metastasis, becomes the well-known mahogany-colored *Bacillus coli.*

It is Dr. Rife's belief that all micro-organisms fall into one of not more than ten individual groups (Dr. Rosenow has stated that some of the viruses belong to the group of the streptococcus), and that any alteration of artificial media or slight metabolic variation in tissues will induce an organism of one group to change over into any other organism included in that same group, it being possible, incidentally, to carry such changes in media or tissues to the point where the organisms fail to respond to standard laboratory methods of diagnosis. These changes can be made to take place in a short period of time as forty-eight hours. For instance, by altering the media – four parts per million per volume – the pure culture of mahogany-colored *Bacillus coli* becomes the turquoise-blue *Bacillus typhosus.* Viruses or primordial cells of organisms which would ordinarily require an eight-week incubation period to attain their filterable state, have been shown to produce disease within three days' time, proving Dr. Rife's contention that the incubation period of a micro-organism is really only a cycle reversion. He states:

> In reality. It is not the bacteria themselves that produce the disease, but we believe it is the chemical constituents of these micro-organisms enacting upon the unbalanced cell metabolism of the human body that in actuality produce the disease. We also believe if the metabolism of the human body is perfectly balanced or poised, it is susceptible to no disease.

In other words, the human body itself is chemical in nature, being comprised of many chemical elements which provide the media upon which the wealth of bacteria normally present in the human system feed. The bacteria are able to reproduce. They, too, are composed of chemicals. Therefore, if the media upon which they feed, in this instance the chemicals or some portion of the chemicals of the human body, become changed from the normal, it stands to reason that these same bacteria, or at least certain numbers of them, will also undergo a change chemically since they are now feeding upon media which are not normal to them, perhaps being supplied with too much or too little of what they need to maintain a normal existence. They change, passing usually through several stages of growth, emerging finally as some entirely new entity – as different morphologically as are the caterpillar and the butterfly (to use an illustration given us). The majority of the viruses have been definitely revealed as living organisms, foreign organisms it is true, but which once were normal inhabitants of the human body – living entities of a chemical nature or composition.

Under the universal microscope disease organisms such as those of tuberculosis, cancer, sarcoma, streptococcus, staphylococcus, leprosy, hoof and mouth disease, and others may be observed to succumb when exposed to certain lethal frequencies, coordinated with the particular frequencies peculiar to each individual organism, and directed upon them by rays covering a wide range of waves. By means of a camera attachment and a motion-picture camera not built into the instrument, many "still" micrographs as well as hundreds of feet of motion-picture film bear witness to the complete life cycles of numerous organisms. It should be emphasized, perhaps, that invariably the same organisms refract the same colors when stained by means of the monochromatic beam of illumination on the universal microscope, regardless of the media upon which they are grown. The virus of the *Bacillus typhosus* is always a turquoise blue, the *Bacillus coli* always mahogany colored, the *Mycobacterium leprae* always a ruby shade, the filter-passing form or virus of tuberculosis always an emerald green, the virus of cancer a purplish red, and so on. Thus, with the aid of this microscope, it is possible to reveal the typhoid organism, for instance, in the blood of a suspected typhoid patient four and five days before a Widal is positive. When it is desired to observe the flagella of the typhoid organism, Hg salts are used as the medium to see at a magnification of 10,000 diameters.

In the light of the amazing results obtainable with this universal microscope and its smaller brother scopes, there can be no doubt of the ability of these instruments to actually reveal any and all micro-organisms according to their individual structure and chemical constituents. With the aid of its new eyes – the new microscopes, all of which are continually being improved – science has at last penetrated beyond the boundary of accepted theory and into the world of the viruses with the result that we can look forward to discovering new treatments and methods of combating the deadly organisms – for science does not rest. (a hope not yet realized in the "accepted world" of cancer treatments, BJF, 2014).

To Dr. Karl K. Darrow, Dr. John A. Kolmer, Dr. William P. Lang, Dr. L. Marton, Dr. J. H. Renner, Dr. Royal R. Rife, Dr. Edward C. Rosenow, Dr. Arthur W. Yale, and Dr. V. K. Zworykin, we wish to express our appreciation for the help and information so kindly given us and to express our gratitude, also, for the interest shown in this effort of bringing to the attention of more of the medical profession the possibilities offered by the new microscope.

1946   Rife's drinking forces him to sell off his lab piece by piece. He is committed for "alcohol rehabilitation."

1948   Drs. Virginia Livingston-Wheeler & Eleanor Alexander-Jackson, micro- biologists in Philadelphia prove that the cancer virus "is in actuality a pleomorphic bacterium."

1949   Dr. Virginia Livingston becomes the head of New Rutgers Presbyterian Laboratory in Newark, NJ.

1949   June 6: Morris Fishbein is ousted by the American Medical Association at its Atlantic City Convention. Reason: years of advertising fraud and fund stealing.

1950   Rife is released from rehabilitation and returns to work. He forms a partnership with John Crane, an engineer/scientist. Crane "re-invents" the Beam Ray and hires Verne Thomson, an electronics expert with the San Diego police force, to help construct the new machines, the new Frequency Instruments.

Rife began to explore the world of living tissues early in the 1920's. To do this he needed a powerful microscope and one that did not destroy living tissues. In CD number four of *Rife Speaks in 2000*, he says:

"I designed and built the first of my hipowered microscopes in 1922. It had a magnification of 17000 and a resolution as high as 9000. Silver nitrite did not suffice as the illuminant for this instrument." (So, Rife explored other forms of illumination like prisms, settling eventually on quartz as the substance for his lenses) Rife continues, "Each individual microorganism had a certain chemical component. Certain chemical constituents would create a color index – an index called 'frequency (wave) of light color index or refraction'".... "The first (frequency) instrument in 1920 was used to determine individuality of microorganisms – primordial cells." (Cells had unique shapes and refracted different colors).

"I designed and built the second microscope in July 1932. I helped them (Drs. Tulley, Rosenow, and myself) see Polio Miletus." (An improved version of the 1932 Instrument, the "Clinical version" was the Frequency Instrument in the summer 1934 clinic).

Rife continues, "I have isolated a great number of these primordial cells.... (The story of my Universal Microscope, written by Dr. Seidel and his assistant, Mrs. Winters, was published in the Smithsonian Report and the Franklin Institute. No other microscope surpassed the Universal."

Work continued on the 1934 Clinical version of the Frequency Instrument after the clinic. The Instrument was improved again in the 1959's so much so that Rife could write in a 1956 letter about the latest version that it was infallible (mistake free) and simple (easy to operate). After reading extensively on Rife, interviewing engineer David Tumey, I am convinced that Rife found a MOR (mortal oscillatory rate) with his Frequency Instrument, a frequency (color) (vibrating) rate that when matched to the frequency (color) of the invading microorganism B. X. or B. Y. , devitalized (killed, destroyed) the microorganism. The true chemical color for Cancer Virus B. X. is purple-red, for Typhoid Virus is Turquoise, *Bacilli coli* virus is dark brown, for Polio virus is reddish brown and for Herpes virus is coral pink.

Royal Rife had initiated a new scientific field: the classification of color of micro-organisms and the non-invasive, painless treatment by an authentic Rife Frequency Instrument, set at the proper frequency (Mortal Oscillatory Rate) the diseases color, that devitalizes the particular diseases microorganism. There was no pain and no destruction of any healthy cells or tissue. Contrast that with one of the staples of 2014 standard cancer treatment, chemotherapy. Chemotherapy drugs that earn millions for drug companies and some doctors, attack every rapidly dividing cell in the body, both cancerous and healthy rapidly dividing cells. They are deadly poisons.

Why did Royal R. Rife's Universal Microscope work in terms of assisting him in finding and experimenting with the B. X. (Carcinoma) virus, curing the cancer without destroying healthy tissue, cells, etcetera..?

The answer is because his microscope utilized natural light (colors that he discovered, that identified different viruses) reflected, and that matched the MOR, the Mortal Oscillatory Rate of the light frequency to match the color of the virus. When the virus was exposed to the matching frequency color of the ray, the virus devitalized (was destroyed).

Why and how did I become interested in Royal R. Rife's life and work?

The answer is that my engineer friend, David Tumey, had introduced me to Royal Rife in his 1990's paper with William Sheline on their recreation of the original Rife Ray Tube.

(That paper is included in Part One, subtopic *A New Light on Cancer,* number 16 of this e-book).

My interview and discussion with David in 2012 which was updated in late 2013 deepened my interest in Royal Rife's work in the discovery of a cure for cancer in 1932. I included Rife's work in my *Called into Life by the Light* series of five e-books and audio books because the overall theme of the series is that Light is a Someone and a Something.

The Ultimate Someone is God, Psychic Energy centered in three Divine Persons, so united as to be One Divine Eternal Being, One God. Light is also a Something in nature, the physical world – the basic physical, empirical stuff of the universe.

The Medicine of Light is one use of light as a something, Rife's Microscopes and Frequency Instruments revealing and then devitalizing, destroying a speck of light, the cancer organism, and thus healing a person's body of a particular form of cancer. All of the most effective and least invasive diagnostic procedures and devices used in accepted modern medicine are light based like the CT Scan, MRI (Magnetic Resonance Imaging), Ultra Sound, X-ray, and Focused Laiser.

It was **not** my purpose in writing this e-book to present a detailed comprehensive account of Royal R. Rife's life and accomplishments in the medicine of light. That has already been amply documented in Barry Lynes' books and a number of other sources. Google Royal R. Rife to see them.

I am not a Physicist or a Bacteriologist – but I do understand the parameters of sound research. I served for two years as the Associate Director of the Applied Educational Research Training Program at the University of Massachusetts during my required full-time residency for my Doctorate in Educational Administration. This University program was one of eighty-four funded by the Federal Government at Universities throughout the United States in the late 1960's in an attempt to educate at the Doctoral level a cadre of School Administrators and Professors who would develop educational practices that had a researched scientific bases rather than on folklore.

My dissertation theme was an attempt to develop a measuring instrument that to evaluate whether or not a particular research training program was meeting its stated goals or objectives. In 1968, my dissertation was chosen as one of the best in my field and included in a time capsule inserted in a cornerstone at the Air Force Academy in Colorado.

I spent forty-six years devoted to educational reform that was scientifically based on child development, especially how children learn. Two editions of my book *Reform of Schooling,* University Press of America, 1993 and 1995 document my national efforts under a special grant from IDEA, the then Education Innovation Branch of the Kettering Foundation. What I advocated in these books is now considered the way to go. Some Charter Schools and "Progressive School Systems" area implementing these "Reforms" like the Pioneer Valley Performing Arts Charter School in South Hadley, Massachusetts.

So, my effort in reporting on Rife's accomplishments was directed toward citing the documented facts of what he did and leave it up to my readers to decide whether they believed the story. What happened to Royal R. Rife's work is not a rare occurrence when one tries to bring about any sort of real change in a major area like medicine or education. Proven educational innovations take an average of fifty years before they are widely adopted. In Rife's case, it has been more than eighty years since he first discovered and demonstrated a cure for some cancers. The Timeline of his life and work presented in this e-book details the opposition he encountered.

Where is Rife's Microscope and Frequency Instrument as of 2014?

We'll present some answers in Part IV of this e-book.

1950   Dr. Irene Corey Diller of the Institute for Cancer
        research in Philadelphia isolates fungus   agents
        from cancer growths. Unknowingly she has replicated
        Rife and Gruner's work. She sets up a symposium in
        New York in order to announce her discovery. It is
        killed by Dr. Cornelius P. Rhoads, the head of
        Memorial Sloan-Kettering Cancer Center. Dr. James
        Hillman of RCA Labs in Princeton. NJ, later confirms
        the Livingston-Wheeler-Gruner-Rife pleomorphism.

1953   Dr. Diller publishes her discovery: *Studies of Fungoid
        Form Found in Malignancy*. Dr. Livingston-Wheeler
        presents her own discoveries to the 6th International
        Congress of Microbiology in Rome. Sep. 10: The
        Washington Post reports. "The New York Academy of
        Medicine immediately discounts the announcement."
        Dr. Rhoads of Memorial Sloan-Kettering Cancer Center
        stops all funds for the Rutgers-Presbyterian Hospital
        Laboratory. The lab is closed, putting Dr. Livingston-
        Wheeler out of business.

1954   Dr. Livingston-Wheeler moves to San Diego, taking a
        job with a clinic. The Committee on Cancer Diagnosis
        and Therapy of the National Research Council
        "evaluate" Rife's discoveries and conclude that "they
        couldn't work." (Please note: never at any point, and to
        this date, no orthodox cancer agency has tested Rife's
        work.)

        Rife, under Crane's insistence, copyrights a description
        of his cancer cure.

1958   Jan: A group of Salt Lake City doctors begin using the
        Rife Frequency machine. In May the Salt Lake City
        Medical Board forces them to stop using it.

116

The California Public Health Dept. holds a hearing. A Frequency Instrument had been provided for testing to the Palo Alto Detection Lab., the Kalbfeld Lab., the UCLA Medical Lab. and the San Diego Testing Lab. All declared that it was safe to use. Result: The American Medical Association Board under the Calif. Director of Public Health, Dr. Malcolm Merrill declares it unsafe and bans it from the market.

1958   July 14. Dr. Virginia Livingston-Wheeler is the first speaker at the 1st International Congress of Microbiology and Leukemia in Antwerp, Belgium. She discovers that the pleomorphism of cancer is widely accepted in Europe while ignored in the United States.

1958   November: After six months of testing Rife's technology, Dr. Robert Stafford of Dayton, Ohio, presents his findings to the Executive Committee of the General Practice Section of the Montgomery County Medical Society of the American Medical Association. The committee is impressed. They set up a research committee from Dayton's most influential doctors.

1959   Dr. Clara Fonti of Milan, Italy "inoculates herself with a bacterial culture of cancer." She grows a tumor, later surgically removed. Thereby proving pleomorphism as a factor in human cancer.

Dr. Livingston-Wheeler meets her neighbor Royal R. Rife.

1959-1960   Dr. Livingston and Rife work together. She arranges for the Institute of Cancer Research in Philadelphia to provide Rife with mice. Their views on pleomorphism are much the same. The only difference is that Dr. Livingston intends to develop a serum while Rife knows the virus disintegrates under his Beam Ray.

117

Dr. Royal Raymond Rife: The Man, His Frequency Instruments, Microscopes, and B.X., The Cancer Causing Microbe

The first CD, in the fifteen CD series of *Royal Rife Speaks in 2000,* was recorded by John Crane in late 1959-1960 when the raid took place on Crane's office. Rife says "I'm 72" (and that would have been in 1960, the year before Crane's trial. Rife had gone into hiding in Mexico by 1961. The CD begins with John Crane saying that this is a message from Royal Rife to Dr. Robert Stafford).

Then Royal Rife speaks:

"This is Royal Rife speaking to Dr. Robert Stafford. I hope if I live long enough to be able some day to shake your hand. What you are doing is a milestone in the field of electronic medicine for the devitalization (destruction) of viruses in the human body. I am 72 years old (1960) and worked over fifty years in this research. You speak of your experimental work on animals. I gave John Crane here last week the data on the pure experimental work on research animals. (John Crane is listening in and verifies that Rife sent the information to Stafford). I never used less than eleven animals – always carry one in "control" uninoculated and the other ten inoculated. It is extremely important, Doctors, that before you inoculate any animal, you put the animal under partial anesthesia because the shock of a needle into an animal as small as a mouse or rat will change their metabolism almost immediately and the change will last for weeks. We have to be sure that they don't die from something else. I never use an animal that has not gone for at least ten days through quarantine – complete isolation. What we wish is the end results. We never know what disease they might have. The adverse conditions that we work under are terrific. When I die, there is a possibility that someone may say 'the old man knew something'. That's all. I worked sincerely and

118

honestly over fifty years on the on the work I gave my life to. My degrees count for nothing. It is only the end results that count. The work you're doing, Dr. Stafford, is marvelous and I appreciate it. The metabolism of a rat is two hundred seventy times more rapid and a mouse four hundred times more rapid than a human being. That has to be taken into consideration. We use a long (sterile) needle directly into the animal. If your inoculant was good, we'll have a tumor which is large in five days. I used a live virus directly from a live breast tumor. It will develop into a mammary tumor if the inoculation was good.

We remove this tumor and find there the exact virus that we have isolated from a human breast cancer. We find there that exact virus we have isolated from the ulcerated breast mass (the cancer we used to inoculate from). We recover from this tumor the exact virus we isolated – we term it B.X. If repeated technically correct, we can reproduce a tumor in the experimental rat from which you can recover the B. X. virus. It's a long drawn out process. It's taken me many years but it has been done thoroughly and well. No slip-ups, no mistakes. But you will not be able to see this virus with your microscope in your lab. As I have stated many times before to my colleagues and associates, the isolation of this organism is a technical proposition. It cannot be seen with your microscope because it is smaller than the wavelength of light. It must be seen with the so-called Rife Microscope. (Even there we do not see the virus itself) but a reflection of it through a series of prisms (that Stafford's microscope did not have). (The reflected) virus has its own particular color, B. X virus reflects red-purple (cancer).

(At this point in CD number one, Rife repeats what he previously said on the importance of proper conditions for selection and use of mice and rats. The stress he was undergoing in 1960 from the American Medical Association and the Food and Drug Administration raid on Crane's office showed in his voice and some repetitions).

He continues with: We do not see the form itself but its reflection by its color index. Different viruses reflect different colors. I devised an instrument that emanates a frequency from this device that is coordinated to the chemical constituents of a live organism (its color frequency) and we devitalize (destroy) it. We recommend no more than two or three treatments a week so that the toxins of the dead materials may be eliminated from the body (between treatments).

1960   John Crane writes and copyrights a manual explaining how the Frequency Instrument is to be used. Dr. Stafford of Dayton suggests that he, Stafford, manufacture and distribute the machine in the USA. Crane decides to license the machine to prevent doctors from changing it, thus failing to get results. Ninety machines are distributed "for research and verification on notarized contracts."

1960   The American Medical Association and the Food and Drug Administration strike. Crane's office is raided. $40,000 in equipment is taken along with all engineering data, research records and reports, pictures off the wall, private letters, invoices, tape recordings, electronic parts. All without a search warrant! Doctors who have the machines are visited and forced to give them up. Ordinary citizens who have begun experimenting personally are threatened. One woman is hospitalized from shock by the American Medical Association raid.

Rife and Crane are arrested and released on bail. Rife, almost 73, unable to handle more   abuse, goes into hiding in Mexico.

1961   Spring. John Crane's trial lasts 24 days. "The records and materials seized are not allowed to be used by Crane in his own defense ... Rife's deposition is not permitted to be introduced." The foreman of the jury is an American Medical Association doctor; the balance of the jury is screened to make sure they have no medical nor electronic knowledge. "No medical reports from the 30's and 40's are admitted. Neither are other doctor's reports. Nor is a Frequency Instrument demonstrated much less admitted into court." The only medical opinion offered by the State of California is from Dr. Paul Shea who had been given a Frequency Instrument by the Public Health Department two months before the trial Shea admits he never tried (it) or made tests to evaluate it. He simply examined it and decided that it had no curative powers and didn't lend itself to investigative use.

Crane is found guilty and sentenced to ten years in prison. Later the State Supreme Court, on appeal, reverses two of the three counts against Crane "because no specific criminal intent had been proven." Crane spends three years and one month in jail. After Crane's imprisonment Dr. Stafford of Dayton is forced to give up his instrument and to give up medicine. A Salt Lake City Doctor's instrument was sabotaged and he was so hounded by the orthodox medical authorities that he commits suicide.

1962   Dr. Livingston has a heart attack. She recovers.

Kefauver amendments to the Food and Drug Act of 1938 grant to the Food and Drug Administration the right to determine if a drug is effective. Safety is no longer a prime consideration. Drug treatment effectiveness and safety is thereby taken out of the hands of the doctor and his patient.

1964   John Crane is released from prison. He begins the fight all over again.

1965   October: Crane submits an application to the Calif. Board of Public Health for approval of the Frequency

Instrument. "The application is made in the name of Rife Microscope Institute," John Crane, owner. The Health Department answers that Crane must first show the instrument to be effective.

Dr. Charles W. Bunner, Chiropractor, agrees to provide "proof of effectiveness." The California Department of Health pays him a visit and forbids him to use the instrument, and present him with a court order to have it destroyed.

Dr. Les Drown, Chiropractor, provides a statement. An American Cancer Society representative subsequently forces him to "sign over" his Frequency Instrument or go to jail. (Rife's cancer discoveries are never patented.) Rife returns from Mexico.

1966   Dr. Livingston and her old colleague, Dr. Eleanor Alexander-Jackson present a paper at an American Cancer Seminar in Arizona. When Dr. Alexander-Jackson returns to Columbia University she discovers that she and her work have been terminated.

1968   Dr. Livingston and her husband open a clinic in San Diego.

1968-1983   They treat over 10,000 cancer patients utilizing her serum and a high immune- building diet. An eighty percent success rate. (The State of California Department of Health has subsequently tried to shut down her clinic. They have also outlawed the use of her serum. Personal communication from the Livingston Medical Center.)

1969   March 4: Rife signs ownership of his microscope over to John F. Crane. It is Crane who preserves all of Rife's work that remains.

1969   Nov. 5-8: Drs. Livingston, Alexander, Diller and Dr. Florence Seibert from the Veterans Administration Research Laboratory in Bay Pines, Florida present a paper: *Microorganisms Associated with Malignancy.*

1970   Oct. 30: Their paper is published.

1971   Rife dies. He has been hospitalized for intoxication. Records show he is given an extra (overdose) of Valium. A mixture of Valium and alcohol is lethal. He is eighty four.

1971   December 23: President Richard Nixon signs a $1.6 billion law to open the "war on cancer."

1972   Dr. Livingston publishes her first book: *Cancer: A New Breakthrough.* She condemns the NCI for its misuse of money and "the use of people as guinea pigs for a 'surgery-radiation- chemotherapy' program dictated by special interests."

1973   The Supreme Court rules that the Food and Drug Administration "can decide without a hearing which evidence it would allow."

1980   "The American Medical Association is found guilty by a U.S. Court of Appeals of 'conspiracy to restrain competition ... New methods of health care have been discouraged, restricted and in some instances eliminated. '"

1984   Dr. Livingston-Wheeler publishes *The Conquest of Cancer.* She warns that most chickens have the cancer microbe.

1985   The Sloan-Kettering Cancer Institute finds the Rife-Livingstone-Wheeler organism (virus) in all blood cultures of cancer patients. They conclude that the organism comes from outside contamination and bury the report.

1985   By this time the National Cancer Institute is spending $1.2 billion dollars annually for cancer. This does not count the monies raised by the American Cancer Society.

1986   Barry Lynes, author of *The Cancer Cure That Worked,* meets John Crane. Crane's willingness to share the facts he knew from his twenty-year (1950-1970) working relationship with Rife, much of it recorded on the many documents Crane had managed to preserve despite the 1938 destruction of the Burnett Laboratory and the 1944 destruction of Rife's records kept by Milbank Johnson, the day before Johnson was to present the Rife Findings to the American Medical Association, made Lynes book possible.

1988   Rife Labs is formed to revitalize Rife's work.

1990   It is estimated that $50 billion dollars have been spent on the "War on Cancer." Twenty percent of this money is spent on actual research. Dr. Virginia Livingston-Wheeler dies.

1996   June: John Crane dies totally destitute in San Diego County. (Personal communication from the Cancer Research Organization.)

1998   May: Nothing has changed as of this writing. Rife Frequency Treatments are illegal except for experimental purposes. It reputedly cures AIDS but the frequencies are absolutely forbidden to be used even for experimental purposes in the United States only. The existence of the Black Field Microscope continues to be denied by orthodox medicine as is the pleomorphism of bacteria/viruses. The suppression of alternative cancer treatments remain in full force and now also includes Hydrazine Sulfate.

Just last year the Food and Drug Administration raided and demolished the San Diego offices of American Biologics whose clinic in Tijuana uses alternate cancer treatments.

How long can this last?

Compiled by A. Walter, 5/98   (16 years ago in 2014)

Dr. Royal Raymond Rife: The Man, His Frequency Instruments Microscopes, and B.X., The Cancer Causing Microbe

What I Learned and Self Help Questions for Part Three

1. After reading/listening to the amended Timeline information about Royal Rife's life, list three things that you learned about him as a person.

2. Why was his Universal Microscope so important to modern medicine?

3. In the United States standard medicine looks at the living body as chemical first and second as electrical.
   Modern Physics sees the living body as primarily electrical. Essentially modern medicine has ignored the electro chemical part of the body. At most   it is tolerated as "alternative medicine/therapies".
   Based on your reading of Rife's clinics and Frequency (Ray) Instruments, how does the focus on a chemical body hurt you if you get cancer?

4. Why are fair, clinically supervised replications of Rife's discoveries, using his microscope, authentic frequency instrument(s) *minus* chemo, and radiation *not* allowed by American Medical Association, food and Drug Administration, etcetera?

Part Four: Royal Raymond Rife: Who? 1999 – 2014

When engineer David Tumey brought me the *Dr. Royal Rife Speaks Again in the Year 2000* set of fifteen CDs on January 27, 2013, we talked about further development of the list of cancers that would be devitalized, destroyed, by a recreated Royal Rife Ray Tube, like the Beam Ray improvement.

He told me that the Federal Government would not approve the technology without ten to fifteen million dollars more of research. Also, this kind of technology still considered to be "alternative" and out of the mainstream. David thought I'd hear on the tapes that Rife himself was arrested for experimenting. His colleagues were arrested, their Rife machines confiscated, and records destroyed. As presented in Part Three, Rife was arrested, exonerated but so broken that he began to drink. He became an alcoholic.

I listened to Rife speak in 1956 on the tapes. He would repeat himself, and inject that he knew that because of the American Medical Association and major cancer research hospitals attitudes toward his work, and as David Tumey said, the huge expense needed to prove his findings with many more trials over time, his treatment for cancer and other microorganisms based illnesses would not be developed.

The large pharmaceutical companies had millions and more to spend on their products and financially supported hospitals and doctors with grant money, free gifts, and percentages of the cost of their products, like the chemotherapy drugs. So, a noninvasive, light-based technology that could help millions of people with various cancers and other serious ailments will probably remain a forlorn hope. Those were David's and even Rife's thoughts. But I think back to the 1980's when there was an article in the National Geographic Magazine on Photovoltaic panels as a son based source of electrical energy.

At the time, the cost of the filaments in the cells was a significant factor but less expensive and more efficient filaments were being developed. The article also reported that an outfit called Mobiltyco, an oil conglomerate had bought up the company doing most of the technology. They managed to delay the process. Thirty plus years later in 2014, Photovoltaic solar based energy is taking off, but still expensive. Yet it is very feasible depending on the latitude (distance from the Equator) and elevation where you live. High priced oil and the "futures" betting where big money outfits and persons bet on the price of oil and manipulate the price irrespective of supply and demand.

The same type of renewal interest in Royal Rife's work is happening in the Twenty-First Century. First of all, the American Medical Association, United States Research Hospitals and United States Pharmaceutical Companies do not have the same combined stranglehold on doctors and hospitals working in France, Canada, Germany, and other European countries. Significant research has continued in these countries using Royal Rife's 1930s-1950s technology from 2009-2014.

Theresa Welsh's Review of *The Cancer Conspiracy* by Barry Lynes (2002 edition, Review written November 2002, Used with permission given October 29, 2014)

The content of the first part of T. Welsh's review is well documented in Part Three of this e-book. I will begin with *The Modern Revival* section of her review. "Today, (2002), there is a renewal of interest in Rife's research, and Rife-inspired machines are being used in Europe to treat cancer and other diseases."

Bernard Fleury's note: That was true in 2002 and is still true in 2014 as I will document later in this part of the book. Can a Rife device actually cure cancer?

"Here is an answer given at the Rife Forum, a web site for European use of Rife technology: Rife claimed that his

128

original machines cured cancer. We have no reason at the present time to doubt this claim but *it has not been absolutely proven."*

Bernard Fleury's note: Rife, himself, admits in his own words that despite all his replications of "cures", more professionally documented "cures" were needed.

"We don't know exactly how the original machines worked and so the modern machines   probably don't work in exactly the same way. Some modern machines have been shown   to have been useful in the treatment of some cancer patients but it would be misleading to claim that they represent an absolute cure for cancer."

Bernard Fleury's note: David Tumey and William Sheline recreated a copy of the Rife Ray Tube in the late 1990s so he and Sheline did know how the Frequency Instrument worked. Dr. Stafford had repeated Rife's experiments during Rife's lifetime. His engineer Harold Leland had given to David the resonators. So David has the original Frequencies. He also now has a non-functioning original Rife Ray Tube. See Part Two, second, fourth, fifth, and sixth pages of our discussion.

Please note: David Tumey's disclaimer at the bottom of the fourth and top of the fifth pages in Part Two.

"My involvement has been in developing electronic hardware on a contract engineering basis. I have never made any claims about the device being intended to diagnose, treat, cure, or prevent any disease or illness."

The Book

Theresa Welsh writes: "While the Royal Rife story is fascinating, Barry Lynes book leaves much to be desired. It is a poorly organized rant against the defamers of Rife that will probably alienate some readers."

Bernard Fleury's note: The first printing of *The Cancer Conspiracy* was in 2000, the same year as the eighth printing of *The Cancer Cure That Worked*. The Conspiracy book was published again in 2002, right after the 2001 ninth printing of The Cancer Cure book.

"Conspiracy" was the focus of **The Cancer Conspiracy**, so Lynes did get polemical especially when he presents chemotherapy!

Theresa Welsh expresses my sentiment as well when she writes, "The main reason to oppose chemo is not that it is painful and expensive, but because it is ineffective."

"Morris Fishbein of the American Medical Association: An Enemy of Health Care For All".

Theresa Welsh's title says it all concerning Fishbein. See the entries in the Timeline about him!

"Billions of dollars have been given to big research organizations with almost no results. You can wonder about that as you read Barry Lynes angry words. I thing Barry Lynes has something important to say. The medical establishment in America has much to answer for."

Detection of Mortal Oscillatory Rates (MORS) in vevo by David Tumey, Engineer

Bernard Fleury's note: David Tumey sent this article to me in 2012. I added it after the 1984 – Summer, First Cancer Clinic using Rife's Technology, when locating a needed frequency was a major time-consuming problem. This article describes David Tumey's contracted engineering role in solving the MOR problem. See Part Three, Timeline 1934 – Summer First Cancer Clinic for the complete article.

January 21, 2008 – Avery Comarow's Cover Story in U. S. News and World Report Magazine on alternatives to traditional cancer treatment drug medicine. Avery writes that "soft alternatives", forms of "energy" medicine like Yoga, Reiki (healing touch), acupuncture, prayer (Bernard Fleury's note: The Holy Spirit is said to manifest himself through fire, light, sensations of heat energy, etcetera), are being tested and integrated with traditional drug medicine. These forms are all considered non-threatening enough, tokenism that standard medicine can live with.

Bernard Fleury's comment: Are not, at least, some of these honest examples of "energy medicine"? They all involve a form of energy that sometimes heals, and all energy both physical and psychic (the inner light) is ultimately light based.

How to Cure Cancer, Time Magazine, Volume 181, Number 12, April 1, 2013. This Cover Title caught my eye while I was looking for a magazine to read in my dentist's waiting room in April 2013.

Wow! At last a cure!

Then in a three line, small font was written, "Yes, it's now possible – thanks to new cancer dream teams that are delivering better results faster by Bill Saporito." I opened to the **Features** (Table of Contents) page.

Pg. 30: *The New Cancer Dream Teams*

Why amassing a huge cast of Ph. D.s and funding them lavishly might just beat the tumors by Bill Saproito. I turned quickly to page thirty.

"A team-based, cross disciplinary approach to cancer research is upending tradition and delivery results faster by Bill Saporito. THE CONSPIRACY TO END CANCER."

At this point I was eager to read the entire article.

The title in very large upper case print reads, "THE HERO SCIENTIST WHO DEFEATS CANCER WILL PROBABLY NEVER EXIST." The Time Article is reporting that there really is no cure for cancer at this time especially when the cancer is advanced. Small victories here and there are reported.

I read the entire article and I invite you, my reader, to do the same at the magazine source listed in the title of this section. The cover title and subtitle are simply not true. Yes, a team of knowledgeable persons with great facilities and plenty of grant money can produce "results" faster than one person working alone on a shoe string.

So far, one year and eight months after the Time Article appeared, where are the "cures" for any one type of cancer?

Much of the teams' work will be in developing "800 drug agents and similar products." What Rife and a number of well known M.D.s and Ph. D.s, engineering professionals demonstrated in the 1939's and some for a while thereafter, is totally missing. The American Medical Association and Food and Drug Administration and major drug companies did their work well, at least in the United States and Canada.

The organization that was started six years ago is organized into six "dream teams" (cf. pp. 34-35 in the magazine) funded by Stand Up to Cancer (SU2C) by entertainment industry figures like Spider-man producer Laura Ziskin who died of cancer in 2011 and Katie Couric whose husband died of cancer in 1993, unhappy with the progress made against cancer. (page 32 of Time Article). They were supposed to produce "results" in about three years. The stated goal was to cure cancer in its principal forms. No complete cures as of the end of 2014 that I can find reported online.

They work in groups, but as Suzanne Somers relates in her book, *Knockout,* surgery (cut), chemotherapy (poison), and radiation (burn) and a host of drugs with terrible and frequent side effects remain as the deadly treatments that destroy more than they "cure".

Preventing Cancer Before It Starts, by Deb

Whittenmore, Winter 2013 issue of Bay State Health. This is a newspaper insert advertising Bay State Health Services in Massachusetts. A patient had ongoing indigestion and pain. A biopsy revealed that the man had very early stage esophageal cancer and he was referred to Bay State for further evaluation and treatment.

Two Bay State surgeons performed an endoscopic mucosal resection, an option available for treating early stage esophageal cancer.

The next step in his treatment was to receive radiofrequency ablation to prevent cancer from returning.

During radiofrequency ablation therapy radiofrequency energy (less than one second) is used to heat and remove targeted tissue. The out-patient procedure takes less than half an hour, requires no incisions, and uses conscious sedation. Risks are minimal and most patients tolerate the procedure well, experiencing mild pain and difficulty swallowing for about a week, and minimal bleeding.

Bernard Fleury's note: The only reason I included this cancer update is because the doctors used a "radiofrequency ablation" to remove targeted tissue. This procedure "burns" the tissue and removes it. It was **not** used to destroy the early cancer. This article continues with "the process (Barrett's esophagus) needs to be found early in order for ablation therapy to even be possible."

This is **not** the frequency which Rife used. His frequency did not "burn" anything. It was vibrational and caused the actual cancer to vibrate and explode! No pain or bleeding. The destroyed tissue was removed from the body by drinking a quantity of water to flush it out.

Electromyography and Nerve Conduction Studies Testing Your Muscle and Nerve Function

I had been having trouble with numbness and pain in both hands for two years and decided in early 2014 to have it checked out. The doctor who specialized in ailments of the hands told me it sounded like Carpal's Tunnel and that I would need a diagnostic Nerve Conduction Test to measure muscle and nerve function. A fine needle was placed under my skin below my thumb and places on my palm an inch or so below the base of several fingers. Mild electrical current was applied to the skin above where the needle was inserted to see how quickly impulses traveled between nerves. The needle allowed the electrical activity in the muscle to be measured. An electromyography wave form appeared on a screen that showed how well my muscles and nerves were working at each site.

My results indicated that I needed Carpal Tunnel surgery in both hands and tri-monthly Cortisone injections at the palm pad just beneath each thumb.

This test used a form of light based technology to diagnose the degree of dysfunction. It is no threat to established medicine, so it is accepted and it works.

Companies in 2014 Promoting Royal Rife Technology

There are a number of companies advertising Rife machines and telling the story of his life. I searched the internet and found three companies that have Rife technology, instruments and/or accessories. I spoke to representatives from all three of the companies and downloaded literature from all three.

I. Rife Videos.com
    (Your Rife Machine History Educational Website)
    This site is part of KE Enterprises and Design. I verified this based on a common Toll-free and Local telephone numbers for RifeVideos.com. and KE Enterprises. They do tell an extensive and detailed story of Royal Rife and his instruments both in print and in their two videos: *The Royal Rife Story* and *Rife–In His Own Words.* My two sources *David Tumey's Conversation on Royal Rife Ray Tube* and the CDs *Royal Rife Speaks Again in 2000* that I used in this e-book basically have the same content as Royal Rife Videos site

(see paragraphs number three to eleven of Rife Videos Home Page). Also The Smithsonian 1944 Report documents in detail Rife's Universal Microscope and Beam Ray Instruments and how they worked. Their two videos would be nice additions to anyone's library who wants to see and hear all about Royal R. Rife's life and achievements.

Resonant Light Technology White Paper

A real rife machine must have 3 parts:

1. A FREQUENCY GENERATOR

A frequency generator (a.k.a. "TENS" or "micro-current" device) emits electrical frequencies. High-quality units are extremely precise and can be programmed by an end-user.

2. A RADIO FREQUENCY "CARRIER"

Electrical frequencies pulsed from the frequency generator are changed to PEMF. In many plasma emissions devices, the signal is amplified and paired with a "carrier" so frequencies travel farther. This provides freedom of movement during use. Other machines use electromagnetic coils instead of a plasma tube and a carrier, so users must be within inches of the device.

3. A FREQUENCY EMITTER

Electromagnetic frequencies are emitted by the device. Plasma tubes can emit numerous higher frequencies, while coils have a stronger magnetic emission.

How does a Rife machine work?

1. A frequency generator sup- plies precise frequencies.

2. The frequencies are amplified and paired with a radio frequency "carrier", referred to as a carrier wave.

135

3. Frequencies are melded with the noble gas and emitted through a plasma on the carrier wave creating an electro magnetic field.

The Research

Studies date back to the 1930's when Dr. Raymond Royal Rife developed a new treatment method that many of the greatest minds at the time believed could be the end to all disease.

While the technology was suppressed for a time, authors such as Barry Lynes (*The Cancer Cure that Worked*); Dr. Nenah Sylver (*The Rife Handbook*); Dr. James Oschman (*Energy Medicine: The Scientific Basis*) and Brian McInturff (*www.electroherbalism.com*) have been instrumental at educating the public about this technology. This has sparked a whole new generation of independent studies and successes.

Experts such as Dr. James Bare, Dr. Anthony Holland at **Novobiotronics** and the research team at **NovocureTM** continue to break new ground for major illnesses such as cancer, adding to the growing list of achievements being realized with this technology.

A frequency timeline

1890 - Dr. Nikola Tesla
Dr. Tesla's work with electricity and energy revolutionizes modern science and the way we approach frequency concepts.

1925 - Dr. Georges Lakhovsky
Dr. Lakhovsky studies cellular oscillation. In 1925 he writes a Radio News Magazine article entitled "Curing Cancer With Ultra Radio Frequencies."

1929 - Dr. Royal Raymond Rife
136

While pushing innovation in microscope technology, Dr. Rife builds a machine that uses Radio Frequencies (RF) to devitalize cancer cells, the "Rife Machine".

1993 - Dr. James Bare
Fascinated by Dr. Rife's work, Dr. Bare builds his own "Rife Machine" prototype. His findings get international recognition from the scientific community.

1996 - Donald Tunney
From Dr. Bare's initial designs, Don Tunney pushes innovation in frequency technology lightyears ahead. He builds a series of modern prototypes that lead up to the golden standard in Rife technology, the PERL (Photon Emission Resonant Light).

2008 - Anthony Holland
Also working from Dr. Bare's designs, Dr. Holland achieves the devitalization of up to 60% cancer cells using frequencies. Visit www.novobiotronics.com to witness his stunning results and please consider a donation to help his invaluable research.

2011 - Novocure
Novocure gets FDA approval for the use of PEMF technology to treat brain tumors. Novocure is in the process of getting further approvals for various other conditions.

About the PERL M+

The PERL M+ is a non-contact device and addresses the whole body in a non-invasive holistic approach. It not only targets the problem area but helps bring the entire body to a level of homeostasis-boosting the immune system, detoxing, strengthening the organs, increasing energy, reducing stress/inflammation and creating an ideal environment inside and outside of the body for optimal health. So the healing can happen deeply and permanently, not just from a symptom based approach.

There is one major difference in so-called "Rife machines" that are on the market: contact versus non-contact devices. The PERL M+ is a radio-frequency ignited plasma tube and non-contact device like the original Royal Rife machine was, which sends the specific frequency and photon on a carrier wave to the targeted pathogen at the cellular level. So it has full and deep penetration. Other plasma tube devices are induction ignited and lack the RF integration and the deep penetration. RF-ignited plasma tube devices are more efficient than the contact devices. They allow all the cells of the body to be treated at the same time. Certain diseases will require that all cells of the body get treated at the same time.

The contact devices, using an electric current as a carrier, will use the path of least resistance, which is the blood flow, to carry the specific frequencies into the body. This makes it slower and does not allow all cells of the body to be treated at the same time. These are not true Rife machines even if sometimes their "trade name" mentions it.

Contact PEMF machines are effective but only at close proximity. As soon as you distance yourself even a little bit from the coil or whatever accessory you use, you lose power (and efficiency) very quickly.

Computer contact and sound devices are lacking precision in their frequency range and you probably know how important that is when you are targeting a specific problem.

Obviously non-contact devices like the PERL M+ have a bigger freedom of movement during the treatment. As long as you are within 30 feet of your PERL M+ you will get the benefits of the frequencies, independently of the fact that you are sleeping, doing the dishes, watching TV or working on your computer. Some conditions may require several protocols that could last a number of hours (3-10hrs) during the day and it is of course more comfortable to get the treatment while being able to move around and continue with your daily activities. This also means that you could treat a group at the same time. It is much easier using it this way with animals.

The technology is based on integrated sound and light used for the purposes of controlling microorganisms (pathogens). It was first developed and used by Dr Royal Raymond Rife. Its principle is based on two basic phenomena occurring in the human body:

Firstly, because cells and organs are electrical in nature, there are many biological interactions that occur at the cellular level when the pulsed electromagnetic field emanates from the PERL M+. It is believed that when the machine is running on any frequency, the body is taking on an electrostatic charge. This process raises the electrical voltage of the cells, which seems to excite the cells in the body and enable them to communicate with each other more effectively. This enhanced communication in turn, assists the body in becoming more balanced–working towards homeostasis. In other words, the PERL M+ is a tool that supports the body in its repair process.

Secondly, based on the premise that all living matter vibrates to a specific frequency, it is known that there is another major occurrence in the body when a specific pathogen resonates with a specific frequency. When this matching resonance of the pathogen and the emanating frequency occurs, the life force of the pathogen is immobilized or devitalized and what we then have is kill off. The receiving subject may then herx or detox.

Waves of the PERL M+ act within a perimeter of 9 meters (30 feet) and will treat all living things at the same time within that perimeter, while not being physically connected to the device. This is one of the great advantages of the PERL M+.

The ProGen 3, the frequency generator for the PERL M+, currently has over 2000 pre-programmed frequency Sets (protocols). So depending on what you are wishing to use it for, there is probably a program – if not several – that you can benefit from. There are some 50 pages of conditions from A-Z with frequencies contributed by other researchers, which can be viewed at www.electroherbalism.com, and going to the CAFL page. We also recommend the frequencies provided by Nenah Sylver, in her Rife Handbook of Frequency Therapy.

This is an amazing video that came out a couple months ago showing cancer cells being destroyed, by Dr. Anthony Holland TEDx Skidmore College. (http://www.youtube.com/watch?v=zXrZSajlZhw)

Resonant Light Technology's equipment is also unique in that you can pair the PERL M+ with up to 3 ProGens. Each ProGen may be used to send a different frequency to the PERL M+, which will broadcast all of them simultaneously via its plasma tube. This reduces session times dramatically while increasing the benefits of each session due to this more "aggressive" frequency approach. This is known as multisignaling.

In summary then, the PERL M+ not only targets microorganisms and regulates the immune system, but it may also drastically reduce pain, harmonize the body, repair tissue, speed up post-surgery recovery, and heal fractured or broken bones. The PERL M+ has a very calming effect on hyperactivity and high stress loads, and is used by many during meditation or contemplation. The effects of PEMF on the cellular level are more than numerous, and include promoting detoxification, enhancing nerve repair, improving circulation, plus easing both depression and insomnia. Ultimately, the immune system becomes healthier, the nervous system relaxes, and bones and joints become stronger.

140

About The ProGen 3

Resonant Light Technology takes incredibly powerful technology and make it secure, accurate and fundamentally easy to use. In November 2018, they introduced the ProGen 3.

A centered **keypad** design with bigger keys and added functionality make for a more tactile, more responsive user experience. You can now **pause, resume, hold, skip** and **loop** any frequency set.

A cleaner **interface** makes navigating menus and running frequency programs a breeze. The larger screen displays all the information you need at a single glance.

The **laser-etched aluminum** casing protects your investment while providing extra RF shielding, keeping your generator unfazed by outside forces for a flawless frequency delivery for years to come.

On the inside, they quadrupled the maximum output to **4,000,000Hz** and increased the storage capacity to **8190 frequency sets**. This allows Resonant Light to include its **complete database of over 2,000 frequency sets** in every new ProGen, giving you instant access to thousands of programs for thousands of conditions. This listing included all the Sets from the Consolidated Annotated Frequency List (CAFL). For more information about the CAFL, you can visit www.electroherbalism.com

The ProGen 3 has two front-facing **accessory ports** that are used to connect a variety of conductive accessories such as gloves, socks, belts and LED lights. Each port has its own power intensity knob giving you maximum control for maximum comfort.

The ProGen can be powered in two ways. By the **PERL connector** for PERL owners or via the Power connector using the included universal power supply. The **micro USB port** allows you to connect the ProGen to a computer for updates and advanced programming via the ProGen Connect software.

The ProGen 3 is a giant leap forward in frequency technology, both inside and out.

Resonant Light Technology's goal in designing the new ProGen was to give people a portable access to all the benefits this technology has to offer, without compromise.

Resonant Light Interview with Dr. James Bare

Dr. Bare is a living legend in the ever-buzzing world of frequency technology. He is bar none the most accomplished and most knowledgeable scientist to pursue Dr. Royal Raymond Rife's research on frequencies. His contribution is of such magnitude that without him, Rife technology simply wouldn't exist today.

Little-known fact, Resonant Light's founder, Donald Tunney, built his very first prototype 23 years ago using Dr. Bare's research manual. He called it the R.B.T., for Rife-Bare-Tunney. This prototype evolved over two decades to become the PERL M+ we know today.

Resonant Light sat down with him for an enlightening talk about all things frequencies.

1. Dr. Bare, can you tell us more about yourself?

Dr. James Bare : "I am a Doctor of Chiropractic and I have had a strong relationship with natural therapeutics most of my adult life. My interest in frequency technologies goes back into my childhood. When I was 8 years old I discovered Morse Code – a form of pulsed electricity to convey information. Later as a teenager I discovered Tesla, Steinmetz, and others, who literally became my childhood

142

heroes. I graduated from Cleveland Chiropractic College of Los Angeles in 1976. Becoming a Chiropractor provided me with an interest in healing using a variety of electrotherapeutic devices. What appealed to me was that these machines were not chemicals in a bottle and importantly they could be used to heal people.

Around 1993, I was introduced to Dr. Royal Raymond Rife and his work. Things completely clicked for me. I was familiar with the concepts of healing, using wide band Radio Frequencies (RF) through the work of Georges Lakhovsky. I also had heard about the early electrotherapy devices where people would literally take "electric showers". Tesla was also involved with some of these early devices. Barry Lynes book on Dr. Rife was instrumental in my deciding that it might be possible to re-create a device that was similar in some respects to that of Rife's. My first instrument was developed and tested in 1994, and when tested on micro-organisms actually worked! There is a long story to all this, but suffice it to say, my first instrument received worldwide recognition! The rest as they say, is history.

I retired in 2015 after almost 39 years of practice but am still quite active with frequency instruments. Some readers may be aware that I am part of a small research group. We are continually pushing envelopes and trying new things. As a part of the improvements made by Resonant Light to their instruments, the discoveries made and research outcomes from our small group are passed onto Resonant Light and utilized to benefit the owners and users of their instruments."

2. How is your work part of Resonant Light Technology?

Dr. James Bare : "Don Tunney, the founder of Resonant Light, was an important pioneer in the industry. In those early years of the mid 90s, Rife's work and name were almost unknown. There were a few frequency instruments on the market; many were ineffective and flaunted having capabilities they did not possess. There was a lot of negativity about all things pertaining to Rife. Some of this negativity came from inside a small group of people that were working with what they claimed were "Rife devices". Needless to say, I ran into opposition from several sources when I first came on the scene.

Don used the internet to bring forth the worldwide respectability and renewal of interest in frequency therapies to hundreds of thousands of people. He was instrumental in encouraging and helping to nurture development of the fledgling resonant frequency therapies community. A short few years later, Don founded Resonant Light Technology and decided to begin manufacturing his own devices. The early Rife instruments were simple and based upon available components. Don soon saw the need for purpose-made components and took the time, effort, and money, to see that they were developed. He also introduced protocols and frequencies for the community that are used to this day in his legacy device, the PERL M+.

Continuous development has occurred over the following decades. Improvements were based upon lessons learned from actual application and new discoveries, which have continuously improved his original devices. New developments in electronics, along with deeper understandings of physiological processes behind the effects, are the driving force of advancement. We are now literally generations removed and improved from that simple early unit created back in 1995.

The PERL M+ is a modern device, based upon more than 23 years of development of my original discoveries. The PERL M+ didn't get as good and effective as it is overnight. A lot of hard work and effort on the part of Resonant Light has gone into making improvements and what are now multiple generations of devices.

144

A great, state of the art device is just one part of the overall aspect to a frequency instrument. Resonant Light Technology is also the industry leader in customer service. Their multi decade commitment to helping their customers effectively utilize their instruments has been critical to the long history of successes the PERL M+ has achieved. As Don used to say "The device is always working" meaning that one must be able to apply it effectively. Don's legacy lives on not just through the devices, but also through commitment to counselling and assisting Resonant Light customers in the use of their devices."

3. Is frequency therapy the beginning of a new era?

Dr. James Bare : "The problem with society worldwide is that we are all taught from the time we are children to utilize chemicals to treat disease. From the time we are conscious, we are told to "see your doctor". We are told this thousands of times every year and that gets repeated for every year of one's life until they die. Same goes with "take this medication or pill" for this condition or that condition. Get yourself a blue pill, get this immunization and so on. It never ends: one cannot read a magazine, turn on a TV or a radio and not be subjected to this constant form of message reinforcement. Then there are the vicious hit pieces on those that would use a non medical method of healing to treat people. There is a multi-billion dollar influence on government and legislation. Those responsible for the constant unending promotion of health through chemicals have a strangle hold on people's consciousness and governments worldwide. The propaganda persists from cradle to grave.

So that being said, such programming is what someone new brings to the discussion when they are inquiring about frequency therapies. They will often filter what is being said through prior experience and the subconscious meme of "health comes from chemicals". But health doesn't isn't just restored via chemicals. There are many other methods of

145

healing that don't use chemicals to heal. Methods such as Chiropractic, Acupuncture, and many different forms of body energy therapies. Yes, these healing disciplines may also utilize naturally based chemicals for treatment such as herbs or food concentrates (vitamins and minerals) but the point is that health doesn't always have to originate with chemicals.

The use of frequency instruments has been around for well over a century. We just don't tend to think of these instruments as frequency devices. Devices like electro-cauterization units and electric scalpels are frequency instruments. Pulsed short wave diathermy used for deep tissue heating, TENS units, ultra sound units, Bio Feedback devices, Micro Current devices, Bone Growth Stimulators, Lasers used for other treatments, such as acne and weight reduction, are all frequency devices. There are many other devices in common usage that depend upon the use of frequencies. Those frequencies often are specific to the production of a desired physiological effect. So the use of frequencies to heal is nothing new, and are in use every minute of every day worldwide helping people recover their health.

The PERL M+ also uses specific frequencies to produce physiologic effects. One major difference is that the PERL M+ produces those effects through an emitted field, without the person being in contact with the device. The PERL M+ has capabilities that often replicate those of several different types of commonly used frequency devices, while also having effects that are unique to the PERL M+. Owning a PERL M+ is akin to owning a whole room of therapy instruments."

4. What is the biggest misconception about this technology?

Dr. James Bare : "There are a lot of urban legends and hype combined with outlandish claims associated with things called Rife. These stories have created unrealistic expectations. Too many manufacturers are putting the word "Rife" on their devices and then promoting the idea that the device is some sort of panacea. There becomes an expectation of quick success. Success, if it comes, can be slow and gradual. All devices are this way. The path back to health is not a straight one, and is why the customer service and counseling offered by Resonant Light are so important."

5. Are there contraindications to using frequency technology?

Dr. James Bare : "The effects of plasma-emission devices are non-thermal. That is, they occur without creating heat. As such, the PERL M+ is very gentle. Side effects would be detox reactions which could manifest as diarrhea, nausea, or general malaise.

The rare person that is overly sensitive to EM fields can use the PERL M+. They should start out slowly with the device and use reduced exposure times in the beginning. Gradually they can increase exposures times as their body tolerance permits. The PERL M+ has helped those with EM sensitivities return to wellness. The fields emitted from the PERL M+ are coherent, which means the fields through the process of entrainment act to organize and synchronize. The fields emitted from fluorescent lights, clock and wall transformers and other electrical devices tend to be non coherent and can act, especially in those with EMF sensitivities, in a disruptive and disorganizing manner to body processes.

Like all devices there are cautions to its use:

- Do not use the device within 36 hours of administration of chemotherapy medications.
- As a simple precaution, avoid using around anyone that is pregnant.

- If the tube is being pulsed, be careful around someone that is subject to seizures. The pulsed light might set off one.
- Do not touch the tube while it is lit. Do not be closer than 10 inches from the plasma tube.
- Individuals with organ transplants or stem cell transplants are advised to avoid frequency devices as its immune boosting effects may be contraindicated.
- Individuals using defibrillators are advised to avoid frequency devices.
- Individuals using pacemakers manufactured before 1992 are advised to avoid these devices due to the pacemaker's inadequate frequency shielding.
- Using an oxygen tank within 20 feet of plasma-emission devices is to be avoided. Oxygen concentrators are OK.
- Generally speaking, frequencies less than 5 Hz are not recommended for prolonged periods of time."

6. Why are some frequency devices using a plasma tube?

Dr. James Bare : "Not all plasma tube devices are the same in the manner they excite the plasma tube. One should not think that the emissions from all plasma tube devices are the identical! The plasma tube as used in the PERL M+ is an energy conversion device. Being based upon my patents, the emissions from the PERL M+ plasma tube are unique. What is emitted from the PERL M+ is a unique and very complex wide band width of emissions. There is visible light (phototherapy) and there is infrared light as well. Then there is an acoustic component that occurs from both a ringing of the tube glass due to the tube being pulsed, but also the air molecules around the tube being excited in a pulsed manner (sound therapy). There are also pulsed oscillating electrical and magnetic fields, both of which produce physiologic effects. Plasma as created by the PERL M+ is a way to affect many different physiologic mechanisms simultaneously.

148

The primary use of plasma emission technology is to target micro organisms and cells. This is done is multiple ways:

1. Destruction
2. Inhibition of growth
3. Activation of immune system
4. Aiding the immune system in discovering and targeting harmful microbes
5. Activation of internal cell protective mechanisms "Heat Shock Proteins"

There is also the subject of "vitality", which used to be known "vitalism". Vitalism is a term the Medical world almost abhors, for it means that their mechanistic, chemical basis of life model is incorrect. Their model is in fact only partially correct. Vitalism is a part of every non-medical healing model. Vitalism is a part of the new and rapidly expanding science known as quantum biology. Basically, the plasma emissions are vitalizing to the body. This occurs through both adding charge to the body cells as a whole, but also (due to the pulsed nature of the signal) entrainment to the signal pulses, which then results in coherence. In coherence, the body's cells and their metabolic processes become synchronized (for lack of a better word). In other words the immune system and other defensive systems start to work in a synchronized manner.

The plasma created by the PERL M+ offers the largest effective range of any plasma device. A general rule of thumb is 30 feet all around the plasma emitter. This has been proven by rifing sessions Don Tunney used to run in a Courtenay warehouse. People would just come and sit; some of them over 50 feet away from the tube. Participants would fill our questionnaires about their experiences and results of these sessions. I have seen a few of these: they were amazing reports! Undoubtedly, the units will produce effects at over 30 feet.

For example: there was a woman living in an upstairs quarters of the warehouse with some sort of arthritis as I recall and she went into heavy detox and began feeling the benefits of the device when these sessions were started. She was a lot further away than 50 feet. It is the unique electrical circuits within the PERL M+ that allows for response at such large distances. Other plasma devices on the market can have manufacturer recommended distances as short as 18 inches for best efficacy. The effectiveness of the PERL M+ at distance from the tube is unmatched by any other plasma device on the market.

Radio Frequency (RF) means the output energy is oscillating as a sine wave at a particular frequency (the carrier frequency). With RF, there is both an Electric (E) and Magnetic (M) component. E fields, as well as M fields both have been shown to produce physiological effects. A pure high voltage output that is inductively coupled to a plasma tube is not oscillating and thus lacks a magnetic component.

An inductive non-carrier unit is missing the ability to produce an entire range of physiologic effects that the M field can produce. Furthermore, there are physiological effects that can be produced by a carrier wave. There is a whole range of these kind of instruments that are used in the field of medicine. An inductive, non-carrier wave device is also unable to produce effects that are carrier wave dependent. An inductive non-carrier wave device is inherently restricted in its ability to create physiological effects, compared to an RF device.

An important fact that is overlooked and often not mentioned by other manufacturers is that absolutely everything that Rife's instrument is famous for was achieved using a plasma tube based device excited with the use of Radio Frequencies. Rife didn't use electrodes and he didn't use high voltage electricity to excite his plasma tube. Rife didn't use electromagnets; he used an RF excited plasma tube that delivered specific frequencies to create the effects he is famous for."

7. *What makes the PERL's 30-foot range even possible?*

Dr. James Bare : "I am going to offer an explanation, and this explanation destroys the **Inverse Square Law** (ISL) argument being used against the PERL by some of your competitors. Perhaps after hearing my explanation, the ISL can be used to contrast those devices whose operation are subject to this law. All devices that are subject to the law have to be used within a few inches of the body to produce best effects. Not 30 feet like the PERL!

There are two key aspects to this explanation.

First, the body is an **antenna** and will actually produce a "gain" to the signal strength via a natural resonance. The best resonant gain is at around 50 MHz, but there is still a very good resonance gain at 27 MHz as well.

This brings up a point, a human body's resonance and gain at 3.3 MHz is relatively very poor compared to the resonance and gain at 27.125 MHz. Due to poor resonance and little to no gain, devices with a 3.3 MHz carrier are subject to the Inverse Square Law and must be used close to the body to maximize delivery of frequencies. The manufacturers in fact recommend their customers use the devices very close (within inches) to the body.

Further the first harmonic of 27.125 MHz is 54.25 MHz; a harmonic of the carrier wave that the PERL produces. This carrier harmonic includes sidebands and this is right at the peak of body absorption.

Second, the human body is a **capacitor** – why one can walk across a carpet and get a shock by touching a door knob. Capacitors of course store energy. In the case of the just mentioned sparking/shock a human body can store thousands of volts of energy!

This all brings us to the method, a subset of what is known as **Wireless Resonant Energy Transfer** (WRET). WRET is currently used to charge different electrical devices especially cell phones, with the device being in proximity to the field of the charging device. Most of the commercial devices using WRET use magnetic fields to transfer energy wirelessly via induction. Induction works only across a small distance and is also subject to the Inverse Square Law. This is where things get all confused. The PERL does not use Resonant Induction to transfer energy.

As is known, the plasma tube converts RF into an intense Oscillating Electric Field. The wavelength of 27.125 MHz is 35.6 feet . This is important, for the effective distance of the PERL is dependent upon the wavelength of the carrier wave. As the body can act like a capacitor and also is very resonant at 27 MHz, the PERL transmits energy to the human body via what is known as **Resonant Capacitive Coupling**.

From Wikipedia on Wireless Power Transfer:
Near-field or nonradiative region – *This means the area within about 1 **wavelength** (λ) of the antenna. In this region the oscillating **electric** and **magnetic fields** are separate and power can be transferred via electric fields by **capacitive coupling**.*

Here is a video showing the use of a 9V battery and 0.1 ampere of current to light an LED array at 30 cm distance using Resonant Capacitive Coupling. This is an impossibility from the concept of the ISL and even via inductive coupling.

https://www.youtube.com/watch?v=5Bs3VBimAPk

Please note that this is the method Nikolai Tesla sought to

utilize in his World Wireless Energy System.

Bottom line, just like Tesla, the PERL uses Resonant Capacitive Coupling. Due to its 27.125 MHz carrier wave can be effective at distances up to 30 feet . It accomplishes this via **Oscillating Pulsed Electrical Fields** (OPEF) emitted by the plasma tube. These fields being pulsed, are then Capacitively Coupled to the body and resonantly absorbed in the form of frequencies to produce physiologic effects at a distance. The Inverse Square Law does not apply!

This is a hugely significant discovery and makes the PERL stand unique among all other frequency devices."

> **8. *Some people have reported being told that radio frequencies cause cancer. What are your thoughts?***

This is purely and simply a form of fear mongering by some manufacturers out there. To be clear… the answer is no. Especially since the effects of the device are non-thermal (no tissue heating occurs).

Some background 27.12 MHz is channel 14 in band radios. There were once millions of these being used. No truckers or others were harmed or have developed cancer from using 27 Mhz. 27.12 Mhz has been allocated by international agreement for use as what is known as an ISM or industrial, scientific and medical frequency. As such 27.12 MHz is used in hundreds of thousands of industrial, scientific and medical devices world wide. 27.12 MHz was once used by Radio Control enthusiasts. Medical devices have safely used this frequency for decades. There are no reports of cancer or harm from the use of 27.12 Mhz.

Can 27.12 MHz make cancer worse? There is no evidence of that. None. Just the opposite in fact…

> **9. *What do you think of PEMF mats for frequency***

153

delivery?

Dr. James Bare : "There are many different types of mats on the market, but in its truest sense, it is a mat with electromagnets that are pulsed at a very low, fixed rate. The effects are general and the output is primarily that of magnetism. Strength of the magnets is low, as well. So in a way, the effects from this go back to the topic of Vitalism. The units also require direct body contact. A useful device, but with limited capabilities. Mats, in comparison to non-contact PEMF devices, lack the following:

- Wide frequency range into the 100's of thousands of Hz. No access to the physiologic responses that come from variable and high range frequencies.
- There is no light component and thus no physiologic effect from light emissions. Some mats try to make up for this with IR emissions and crystals. However the light from a plasma tube is very wide band and does include IR (includes FIR).
- The Electrical field is extremely weak, compared to a plasma unit. Cannot produce the physiologic effects that depend upon E fields."

10. *Any tips for people looking to buy a device?*

Dr. James Bare : "There is so much hype on the internet, people are confused. In my opinion, one big problem to overcome is that people tend to go with what others are using. The public just gives up at some point and go with a place that seems safest to both them and their investment. Regardless that something else may be vastly superior, they will choose an inferior product every time if that product has a large number of users. That also applies to the device being talked about a lot on the lists.

Is there some sort of research that actually shows an effect of the device upon cancer and infectious micro organisms?

Most devices have nothing except to claim some relationship to Rife. All sorts of claims and implied action are made with no real proof. There are plasma devices on the market now that are partially based upon an old Rife instrument, but it is not that old Rife instrument.

When considering a device, most devices on the market have one or maybe two primary attributes that are used for healing. Maybe they use light, or magnets, or use electrodes for example. The PERL M+ is like having multiple types of devices in one. It simultaneously produces audio waves, electrical fields, magnetic fields, and light. Furthermore, the ProGen can be used as a contact device with conductive accessories.

The PERL M+ has supporting published research that is publicly available and shows efficacy. If a manufacturer claims there is research on their device, has that research been made public? Not just claims, laboratory proven publicly available documents. The PERL M+ being a Rife/Bare device is the only device on the market that has shown to the public actual results of its use on cancer cells, had case studies published, has multiple published and presented papers on its use, and even has video online for people to see for themselves. There are many others claiming research but where is their data?

Another consideration is that Resonant Light Technology has a 23+ year history of producing devices. How long has the other manufacturer been around? There is no other company making plasma emission devices that has been in business as long as Resonant Light Technology. There are literally thousands of instruments that have been produced by Resonant Light which have positively affected the lives and health of tens of thousands of people world wide. That says a lot about the company's commitment to their customers needs, the quality of the devices they are building, and most importantly the efficacy of the devices they make."

PEMF – What is it good for?

Imagine a future in which a single device:

- Vitalizes and supports your body without side effects
- Speeds recovery from injury, illness and surgery
- Reduces stress and promotes good sleep
- Reduces pain and inflammation
- Kills harmful bacteria, viruses, parasites, flukes, fungus, mold and more
- Can aid the body's systems when fighting major illness

Now imagine that it is affordable, easy to use, and accessible to you today.

PEMF, or "Pulsed Electromagnetic Field" therapy uses specific electromagnetic frequencies to target and affect cells and microorganisms within a user's body.

Some frequency ranges you may recognize:

- Radio (such as those that are sent to your FM radio),
- Sound (anything your ears can hear)
- Light (anything your eyes can see)

The right frequencies can kill a pathogen like sound can shatter a glass.

Not all frequency ranges are suitable for use on living organisms.

Reputable manufacturers remain within legal medical ranges and have safety systems to disallow frequencies such as those below:

- Microwave (the frequencies your microwave oven

uses)
* Ultraviolet (the damaging part of the sun's spectrum)
* Gamma Ray (emitted during radioactive decay)

Studies

Exhaustive studies by such experts as Dr. Royal Rife and Dr. Nenah Sylver have uncovered comprehensive lists of frequencies that target particular pathogens or organs in order to help the body fight disease and recover more quickly.

These lists of frequencies are freely available to those who have programmable equipment to be able to utilize them.

Further studies have utilized a variety of PEMF devices to determine the efficacy when used with particular afflictions. These studies have shown success for such issues as those in the following list. To learn more about the literature used, visit www.pubmed.gov and enter the PMID number. These were chosen from thousands of available scientific journals and abstracts on PEMF.

Note: The details below are informational only. We are not suggesting that any device we sell can be used to cure, treat or manage these, or any other disease, malady or issue. We are simply providing a list of clinical successes for your interest.

Bernard Fleury Comment: Note the Disclaimer Wording. The Medical Establishment, even in Canada, still views all of Rife's machines and therapies **at most** as complementary treatments in addition to standard cancer treatments, cut (surgery), burn (radiation), and poison (chemotherapy).

List of Afflictions

PEMF-Is good for:

Arthritis:
* Conclusion of study: "...conclusively shown that PEMF not only alleviates the pain in the arthritis condition but it also affords chondroprotection, exerts anti inflammatory action and helps in bone remodeling ..."
* PMID 20329696
* Worth noting – "also estimated the median lifetime costs (i.e., 25 years following a diagnosis of [Rheumatoid Arthritis]) of RA to be $61,000 to $122,000 (U.S. 1995 dollars)"
(source
http://www.cdc.gov/arthritis/basics/rheumatoid.htm)

Cancer: (see Pancreatic Cancer victory with PERL-M White Paper
* Conclusion of study: "Together these results demonstrated that PEMF exposure significantly increases the anti-tumor effect."
* PMID: 22761760
* Worth noting: "New drugs often cost $100,000 or more a year... and insurers differ on how much they cover"
(source
http://usatoday30.usatoday.com/news/health/story/health/story/20%2012-02-27/Cancers%C2%ADgrowing-burden-the-high-cost-of-care/53271430/1)

Device safety:
* This study covered the safety and efficacy of a new device combining radio frequency and low-frequency pulsed electromagnetic fields (RF with PEMF).
* "The results of this study show that the combination of multipolar RF [Radio Frequency] with PEMF is a safe, effective, and painless approach to treat facial rhytides and is suitable to answer the demands of patients for safe treatments without pain or downtime."
* PMID: 23135079

Erectile dysfunction:
- Conclusion of study: "Recovery and improvement of the erectile function were achieved in 85.7% of patients ..."
- PMID: 17882824
- Conclusion of study: "... beneficial effect was recordable in 70-80 % of the patients ..."
- PMID: 8819933

Fibromyalgia:
- Conclusion of study: "Low-frequency PEMF therapy might improve function, pain, fatigue, and global status in FM patients."
- PMID: 18080043

Osteoarthritis:
- Conclusion of study: "The results suggest that non-thermal, non-invasive PEMF therapy can have a significant and rapid impact on pain from early knee OA and that larger clinical trials are warranted."
- PMID: 22451021

Osteoporosis:
- Conclusion of study: "After 12-week interventions, the results showed that PEMF increased serum 17B-estradiol level, reduced serum tartrate-resistant acid phosphatase level, increased bone mineral density, and inhibited deterioration of bone microarchitecture and strength."
- PMID: 19080282
- Conclusion of study: "The data suggest that properly applied PEMFs, if scaled for whole-body use, may have clinical application in the prevention and treatment of osteoporosis.
- PMID: 2195843

Stroke:
- Conclusion of this study: "Preliminary data suggest that exposure to a PEMF of short duration may have implications for the treatment of acute stroke."

- PMID:17892036

Wounds-Ulcer:
- Conclusion of study: "...is a safe and effective adjunct to non-surgical therapy for recalcitrant venous leg ulcers."
- PMID: 19008935

See specific studies for each of the afflictions listed on Resonant Light Technology site.

PEMF Machines vary in price

Before deciding what a "good price" on a PEMF machine is, please consider the following:

- Family **health care costs exceed $20,000** in 2012 (for a family of four in the United States.

- Hospital stay costs averaged around $33,000 in 2010 (prices doubling since 2000) http://bit.ly/14VLv2A

- **PEMF devices range from $300 to well over $30,000**
  For **$300**, users receive a non-programmable device preset for particular conditions. They are small and easy to use, but do not penetrate as deeply as the higher priced devices, which generally have more power.
  For **$5000,** get a programmable non-contact device that allows free movement of multiple users within 30 feet due to a "carrier frequency". They are easy for non-technical users, but can be damaged due to an external plasma tube (replaceable).
  For **$30,000,** purchase a programmable device that offers biofeedback and FDA approvals, but is quite complex for most users.

The best decisions are based on what the device will be used for and the amount of use the buyer expects to get out of it over a period of years. Don't spend $30,000 if all you have is the occasional sore muscle, and don't purchase a $300 unit if you want to target a virus.

FDA PEMF Approvals

FDA has approved PEMF for a number of uses, including:
- 1979 – Healing of non-union fractures
- 1998 – Urinary incontinence and muscle stimulation
- 2004 – Cervical fusion patients at high risk for non-fusion
- 2006 – Treatment of depression and anxiety
- 2011 – Brain cancer

Resonant Light Technology's PEMF Device – the PERL-M

Research
- Compiled more than 15,000 weeks of data
- More than 2,000 participants
- Thousands of independent studies also available on PEMF

The Company
- Manufacturing PEMF devices since 1996
- Made in Canada
- All units fabricated to medical standards

PEMF Product Details
- **Easy** to use – just follow the prompts on the screen
- **Pre-preprogrammed** with professionally created standard or custom frequency protocols
- **Programmable**, so you can enter your own customized frequencies and protocols as supplied by Resonant Light or other industry experts
- **Non-contact,** 30 foot range provides easy utilization by multiple users and free movement during

operation
- **Quality-** Over 90% of the products built by Resonant Light Technology since 1996 are still operational today!

More Information

To speak with an expert and get all of your questions answered with no cost or obligation, call: 1-250-338-4949 or l-877-338-4949 (toll free in North America.

- Web: www.resonantlight.com

- Email: info@resonantlight.com

- Read the Pancreatic Cancer Victory with PERL-M. Resonant Light Technology was not involved in the case study writing even though the end user purchased the device from them and received support from them. (Edna Tunney, November 7, 2014.)

Pancreatic Cancer Victory with PERL-M!

Pancreatic Cancer is one of the most difficult cancers to put into remission.

In the case of the patient named E. S., a big 4cm. tumor was found in the pancreas next to a major artery. This meant the only **Standard Treatment** available was chemotherapy. With a tumor of that size, and without surgery as a possibility, chances of survival were less than 10%. (Statistic from American Cancer Association [2])

"The average lifespan of the patients is six months after they were diagnosed…these tumoral cells are largely resistant to chemotherapy and radiotherapy, while having a strong potential for remote invasion. (Le Chapellier, B. Matta, *Journal of Cancer Therapy,* p.

461[1])

Chemotherapy was started right away, and E. S. was found to be tolerant and receptive in the original four rounds of the treatment, so an additional three rounds were added. This caused the tumor to shrink to 1.2cm.

Bernard Fleury's Comment: The 4cm. tumor shrank to 1.2cm. after ~~eight~~ *seven* rounds of chemotherapy! ~~Eight~~ *seven* rounds of destroying not only cancer cells but also every other rapidly dividing cell in E. S.'s body!

While shrinkage was a good start it was not enough.

Dr. Le Chapellier and Dr. Matta recognized the dire outlook for this patient using only standard treatments, so they researched a variety of alternatives.   After studying clinical evidence, historical studies and personal accounts of success, it was determined that a **"Rife machine" may provide the results they were looking for.**

Doctors Matta and Le Chapellier were fortunate that works published by Dr. Rife, John Crane, Dr. Bare and Dr. Holland all showed promise with this modality. They also noted that:

> *"The choice of this kind of complementary treatment is best carried out as soon as the pathology is diagnosed and thus before chemotherapy starts".* (Le Chapellier, B. Matta, *Journal of Cancer Therapy,* p. 464 [1])

Bernard Fleury's Comment: So why did Drs. Matta and Le Chapellier not go to the PERL-M Rife Machine before chemotherapy?   Use a non-invasive, harmless, painless intervention instead of chemical poison!

E. S. began treatment with the PERL-M (a Resonant Light Technology device) on October 4th, 2013 under the studious eyes of Dr. Le Chapellier and Dr. Matta at the

Soissons General Hospital in France.

In the first week, E. S. started to notice improved sleep, lessening of diabetic challenges and an increased feeling of wellbeing. By November 7th there was no change in tumor size, but there was a slight "edging" of the tumor.

A CT-Scan on November 17th showed that the tumor had shrunk to the point of being indistinguishable – an extremely significant change in such a short period of time (and a huge win for E. S.) On December 9th further testing confirmed the absence of any cancer on the pancreas.

> *"Thus the conclusion of this unique case study is that a non-invasive bio-electromagnetic treatment, complementary to chemotherapy, applied for two months by means of a PERL device equipped with a confined plasma tube, (a tube emitting EMF frequencies according to Rife-Bare technology), and whose carefully chosen emissions were tuned by a personalized follow-up, caused a disappearance of the patient's tumor associated with a regression of secondary infiltrations,* **constituting an undeniable victory over the pancreatic cancer.*** *(Le Chapellier, D. Matta, Journal of Cancer Therapy,* p. 466 [1])

Because pancreatic cancer is one of the most difficult cancers to put into remission with existing treatments, the results of Dr. Le Chapellier and Dr. Matta's step in the fight against this terrible disease was extremely significant. It is fortunate for everyone impacted by cancer that these doctors had the fortitude to step outside of the standardized tools and delve into options considered "alternative" by their peers.

Bernard Fleury's comment: The "bolding" is mine. Even in France, where they were at least able to do this study at all, they still are doing "alternative therapy" that had to follow the conventional chemotherapy rather than an acceptable and preferable therapeutic protocol!

We will watch the work of these doctors closely as they continue on their quest, and will do our best to share any updates through our newsletter.

-**Written:** June 3, 2014

-**Want updates?** Sign up to receive our newsletter at www.resonantlight.com.

-**The PERL-M is not sold in Canada for human therapeutic use.**

References

[1] Pierre Le Chapellier, Badri Matta, *Journal of Cancer Therapy,* 2014. 5. 460-477: *Is Victory over Pancreatic Cancer Possible, with the Help of Tuned Non-Invasive Physiotherapy? A Case Study Says Yes.*
http://www.scirp.org/journal/PaperInformation.aspx?PaperID=45182#.U4dqzsZVtbw

[2] *American Cancer Association* http://www.cancer.org http://www.cancer.org/cancer/pancreaticcancer/detailedguide/pancreatic-cancer-survival-rates

Open Access Library (No permission needed here)

Scientific Research

Is Victory over Pancreatic Cancer Possible, with the Help of Tuned Non-Invasive Physiotherapy? A Case Study Says Yes.

Author(s) Pierre Le Chapellier, Badri Matta

Abstract

Could the conventional treatment of pancreatic cancer effectively be supplemented by a low level and non-invasive bio-electromagnetic treatment?

Bernard Fleury's Comment: How powerful the cut, burn, and poison lobby is even in France!

A case study, based on the regular exposure of a patient to an electromagnetic field, EMF, emitted by a Rife-Bare technology device, suggests so. The plasma confined in a tube of this apparatus emitted radiofrequency solitons. These low level emissions were modulated by an "audio" frequency generator, pre programmed for the treatment of this disease. After less than two months of exposure to these EMFs, the tumor completely disappeared in approximately two weeks. The explanation of the action mechanism includes a physics aspect relating to the properties of the dissipative soliton which is emitted-absorbed by any non-linear system, a biophysics aspect relating to the coherent structuring of the cellular bath by incident solitons, and finally a biological aspect. The latter is characterized by a critical resonance frequency leading the "*unicellular*" tumoral cell to adopt a self-destructive behavior. On the other hand EMFs with low level solitons have no effect on the tissues of complex multicellular organisms.

Bernard Fleury's Comment: They do not destroy other non-cancerous, healthy tissue like chemotherapy does.

Dr. Rife's Ultimate Rife Machine

Introducing the Rife Machines:

Dr. Rife invented the Rife Machine and helped thousands of people around the world recover from serious diseases including cancer using his Rife frequency devices.

NEW! Rife Machine Professional 2013 CLINIC
Carrier Wave, Radio Frequency switchable Keyboard, Multiple Storage Banks, Dual Frequency. Based on the Original Rife Machine Electronics Clinic or Personal use Rife Machine

Rife Ultimate Machine version 2012/2013
Powerful 16v 4.5 Amp Machine. Easy to use Simple Menu, Plug in and Go – One Million frequencies, 24Mhz Quartz Crystal. Our Bestseller. More than 10,000 machines sold

Bioresonance, by Dr. Rife
The Original Dr. Rife Bioresonance machine. Twelve Volt Output, 2 Amp Cost Effective Budget Rife Machine

With over 15,000 users in Europe and the world, the Rife series now include the "Professional Rife Machine": Powerful, affordable, and suitable for both Clinic and home use.

Higher Amps, Higher Current, Carrier Wave and a keyboard edit menu system, just to name a few new features.

We pride ourselves in sourcing only the highest quality parts from Microchip Devices USA Rife Digital Professional is made under license by Rife Digital Germany. You can have the same positive experiences as Dr. Royal Rife, using this modern Electro-Therapy 'Rife' technology.

Dr. Royal Rife investigated the cause of many diseases including cancer. Dr. Rife used the most advanced microscope in the world to identify the existence of a Virus that he believed was the sole contributor to all cancers. This microscope was the most powerful of its time, and was invented and constructed by Dr. Rife himself; for the sole purpose of locating the Virus that contributed to Cancer...

The birth of the Rife Machine was to be the solution to elimination of this Virus, and Rife performed successful Rife Machine treatments with many patients over the years. This was verified by the U.S.C. Medical School Special Medical Research Committee. USC-0292E41- Page 1203 (b)

The Rife Machines

The Rife Professional Series use specific frequencies from the 3500 frequency list book to stimulate an altering of bioresonance in the cells, reversing the change caused by the disease. Transmitting these frequencies over the same electrodes (straps) over a period of time generates healing signals that have the curative effect. With this method of treatment, practitioners claim to be able to detect and cure a variety of diseases and addictions without drugs.

Used successfully in Germany for more than sixteen months, and with over 15000 users, The Rife Digital Professional series is a German model which is now available to the United States of America. The Rife Digital Professional specializes in running all of the Bioresonance frequencies pertaining to Dr. Rife's original machine. It is a higher powered device using 16v DC, 4500ma, averaging an output of about fifteen volts and one million Hertz frequencies to the body. This model comes into alignment with the standard industry Rife Machines now available for many thousands of dollars more, Rife Digital Professional now incorporates Carrier Wave and Radio Frequency Switchable options to name a few new features.

The Previous 2009-2012 Rife Digital models are now being superseded by the new Rife Digital Professional 2013 device. This model is much easier to use, with simplified easy program keyboard, pause and play function, essential for those bathroom breaks, special comfortable straps designed for use on hands and feet, direct connect silver button on the straps for 100% conductivity to the healing frequencies.

The Rife Digital Series

- The Rife Machine for treatment of all types of disease and related symptoms:
- Rife Digital Professional is the most powerful Rife Machine in the series.
- The Rife Digital Series has output to four straps which can be worn on both feet and hands,
- Use the device for treatment of two people simultaneously.
- We only use quality components manufactured by Microchip Devices USA
- China Parts are not used in the Rife Machine itself. All parts are sourced from Digikey USA
- Please e-mail Dr. Peter Williams on the contact page for a discount on the
  Professional Model.
- Rife Digital is the best Rife Machine available today.
- Please click INFO below for more detailed information.

Rife Digital Bioresonanz

- The Original Rife Digital Series
- Fully Programmable and Utilizes Bioresonance treatment frequencies
- 1Mhz, 20MHZ Quartz Crystal, 10-12 Volt model, 2000 MA
- 50% Duty Cycle with 100% Positive Offset
- USA manufactured chipsets, by Microchip Devices USA
- All Countries Power Supply Adapter (US110v-230/240/250v)
- Idle Mode, Program Mode, Run Mode and Sweep Mode available

Purchase Rife Digital Bioresonanz if you wish to own a Rife Machine at a budget price.

Rife Digital Ultimate

The Worlds' Most Powerful Rife Machine

- "Ultimate" has more than double the Amperage of the Rife Digital Bioresonanz
- Fully Programmable Rife Machine With Equivalent Power of Industry Standard Rife devices
- Utilizes Bioresonance treatment frequencies
- Power Rating: 16v-DC, (Ultimate model has 35% more Power than Rife Digital Bioresonanz)
- Power Adapter Rating: 4500ma,(Ultimate Model has 125% x more Amp Capacity)
- Rife Measured Voltage Output ~14v (Use only Oscilloscope to measure voltage output)
- 50% Duty Cycle (Standard)
- 100% Positive Offset
- DAC Digital Accuracy
- RF Frequencies using CW impedance
- LCD display gives accuracy up to two decimal points. (0999.99Khz)
- Frequency Range: 0000.01Khz-0999.99Khz (=1MHz)
- Lab tested Pure Square Waveform on all Rife frequencies
- Harmonics: Harmonic Waveform periodic on 100% of Frequencies
- Uninterruptible Program Sequences
- Automatic function plus manual over-ride
- Square Wave Output
- Two Strap Connectors for the hands
- Two Strap Connectors for the feet
- USA manufactured chipsets, by Microchip Devices USA
- All Countries DC Switching mode Power Supply Adapter (US110v-230/240/250v)
- Idle Mode: Default Mode, Rife Digital waits for your

instructions
- Program Mode: Press P to Program 10 Frequency Ranges
- Run Mode: Press Run to run frequency full time
- Sweep Mode Press Sweep to Run a Frequency Set at intervals of 10 minutes per Program

Purchase Rife Digital Bioresonanz Ultimate model if.....

(1) You wish to use this Higher Power output for treatment of more serious disease.

(2) You require a Rife Machine that can deliver the higher power of industry standard devices

(3) You prefer Rife Digital to run all the frequency sets for you, automatically

(4) You need DAC Accuracy combined with RF Frequencies using CW Impedance

(5) You need the Larger 24Mhz Quartz Crystal Core.

Rife Digital Professional

- "Professional" has more than double the Amperage of the Rife Digital Bioresonanz
- Fully Programmable Rife Machine With Equivalent Power of CLINIC Standard devices
- Easy to Use and Program Keyboard. Enter frequencies quickly and easily.
- Utilizes Bioresonance treatment frequencies
- Power Rating 16v-DC, Ultimate model has 35% x more Power than Rife Digital Bioresonanz
- Power Adapter Rating: 4500ma, (Professional model has 125% x more Amp Capacity)
- Rife Measured Voltage Output – 14v (Use only Oscilloscope to measure voltage output)
- 50% Duty Cycle (Standard)

- 100% Positive Offset
- DAC: Digital Accuracy
- RF Frequencies-Dr. Rife's Original Machine. Button Switchable
- CW Frequencies-Dr. Rife's Carrier Wave. Button Switchable
- LCD display with more menu options
- Frequency Range: 0000.01Khz-0999.99Khz (=1MHz)
- Lab tested Pure Square Waveform on all Rife Frequencies
- Harmonics: Harmonic Waveform periodic on 100% of Frequencies
- Square Wave Output
- Two Strap Connectors for the hands and feet.
- Two Straps now connect directly to machine (No Y Junction required)
- USA manufactured chipsets, by Microchip Devices USA
- All Countries DC Switching mode Power Supply Adapter (US110v-230/240/250v)
- Standard Sweep, Standard Run,
- PULSE Sweep and Run- New feature which builds power output for one second and Pulses Frequencies into the body
- Convergence Sweep-Runs Two Frequencies simultaneously on the full Million program mode
- Super Sweep-Runs all million frequencies from 0–1 million Hz
- Three Multiple Group Settings. Put Multiple programs in for different people or multiple disease treatments
- Clinic Standard Device. Key in all your patients programs prior to their arrival for treatment.

Purchase Rife Digital Professional model if…..

(1) You wish to use the Higher Power output of the new PULSE feature

(2) You require multiple programs prerecorded for varying disease treatments

(3) You prefer the simplified Keyboard Input facility

(4) You Wish to Switch between Radio Frequencies and Carrier Waves (Rife Original versus Rife later models)

(5) You wish to experience every frequency from zero to one million via Super Sweep

(6) You require the DUAL frequency output of the Convergence Sweep Mode

(7) You need the Larger 30Mhz Quartz Crystal Core.

"Rife Digital Professional Series: The '2013 Rife Machine' was born from Dr. Royal Rife's discoveries: A machine that provided the exact frequencies produced by Dr. Rife's original Clinic model"

About Rife Digital:

Rifedigital.com supplies the world market with the most recent Rife technology. Designed in Germany and distributed throughout United States of America, Canada, Australia, Europe, England, Africa and South America.

The Rife Digital Professional Series are the most advanced Rife technologies available, allowing the user full control of the frequencies desired to heal.

The accompanying 3500 Disease Frequency book outlines thousands of frequencies available to program into your Rife Machine.

Twelve Months Warranty applies to all Rife Digital Machines. Our Service center is in Florida, and Seattle for West Coast. Accessories such as straps and cables have a limited 60 day Warranty. Wholesale and Re-seller Discounts apply to bulk purchases of Rife Digital. Please contact Customer Service for a quote.

Rife Digital sell Rife Machine's world-wide and the average time for postage is three to four days.
Shipping within the United States is faster: two to three days.

Dr. Peter Williams: The Man Who Developed Rife Digital

Bernard Fleury's Comment: The man who developed Rife Digital, the machines, and the website. He is a man who has given much of his career to Rife based theory and technology. His biography taken from "About me" on LinkedIn follows. It is a great example of how Rife lives on in 2014.

Dr. Peter Williams graduated in Medicine from the University of Oxford, United Kingdom in 1970, receiving a Bachelor of Medicine, Bachelor of Surgery (BM BCh). In 1971 Dr. Williams returned to Northern Ireland and worked as a senior Consultant Physician in Acute Medicine at the Whiteabbey Hospital Newtownabbey, Antrim, Northern Ireland for more than twelve years. He then worked in a private clinic in Belfast until 1998 before retiring from Mainstream Medicine and focused on the new forms of Electro Medicine as prescribed by Dr. Royal Rife. Dr. Williams worked with alternative therapy clinics in London using Rife Machines to treat people for various diseases which included cancer. He then moved to Florida in 2007 and had been working with alternative therapy at various clinics within the United States for more than a year. He traveled to Germany in 2008 and with some prominent electrical engineers developed the Rife Digital series based on the original schematics of Aubrey Scoon, a close friend and engineer who reverse engineered an original Rife Machine made by Dr. Rife. In 2008 Dr. Peter Williams set up a manufacturing plant in Freiburg, Germany with some prominent engineers, and began producing the Rife Digital

174

series.

Dr. Peter Williams developed the Rife Digital which shared identical features to the more expensive Rife Machine models, and also used the same frequency ranges for healing treatments. The focus was always the highest quality machine but to also keep the price within the budget of most people who needed treatment, but could not afford spending thousands of dollars. What is important to Dr. Peter Williams was to develop an affordable Rife Machine that people could use to treat and heal serious disease conditions.

In order to make the Rife Machine cost effective, Dr. Peter Williams moved the assembly process to Asia, however all components continued to be sourced from Texas Instruments and Microchip Technologies in the United States. Germany continues to develop the new Rife Technologies, and to supply the main circuit boards for the Rife Machines.

Dr. Peter Williams has interests and experience in electro medicine, mind-body energy medicine, and uses methods of electro medicine in his alternative medicine practice. He lives in Florida, United States where he finds his regular Yoga practice to be the most delightfully grounding aspect of his day.

Dr. Peter's current focus is on the development of Rife Machines using the latest in microchip technologies from Silicon Valley in order to produce a powerful Clinic model of **Rife Digital Series**.

Part Four: Royal Raymond Rife: Who? 1999 – 2014

What I Learned and Self Help Questions for Part Four

1. Based on your reading/listening to Part Three, which of the two Rife Frequency Instrument companies listed in Part Four seems to be Royal Rife authentic?
   Or are they equally authentic?
   Cite your evidence.

2. Standard USA Medical Practice especially with regard to a rigid belief in monomorphism versus pleomorphism has effectively blocked accurate information about Royal Rife and his machines.
   Why does the medical establishment cling to monomorphism?
   How does this rigid belief affect the kind of cancer treatment that is accepted and available?

3. What evidence did you find in the advertisements of the two Frequency Instrument companies and the Pancreatic Cure article that the war against Rife technology is alive and well in late 2014?

Summary

The Mind-Body-Spirit Connection In The Medicine of Light

Part One:

The Importance of Seeing

In the Forward to Jacob Liberman's book, *Light-Medicine of the Future,* John Ott, a pioneer in the field of photobiology, asks the question "Are we to totally discount our own abilities to see, hear, and feel our everyday experience, trusting only the findings of others who differ from us in their view of reality?"[1]   The "real" is often hidden beneath the exceptional. The optical illusions researched by Goethe were accurate illustrations of the behavior of light. We must be open to new insights. Present day scientific methods are not eternal. They do not have the final answer and so cannot be allowed to be an *absolute* norm for what is scientific.

The Human Photocell

That the human body is a living photocell, energized and controlled by light entering the eyes, is one of Liberman's basic and innovative assumptions. (xxv) Once this light enters the body it has a profound effect on both our physiological and emotional functioning as well as the development of our awareness. Our lives are truly dependent on the sun and the small portion of its electromagnetic waves that reach our planet. The approximately one percent of these waves which reach us and are visible, are essential to proper human functioning and evolution.

The Pineal: "Seat of the Soul"

The Pineal, which in humans, is a small pea sized gland located deep in the center of the brain between the two hemispheres and behind and above the pituitary gland, was considered in the early Twentieth Century to be vestigial like our tonsils, with no real purpose. It is now believed that the pineal is the body's master regulator, receiving light activated information from the eyes by way of the hypothalamus. It then transmits this information to the rest of the body telling whether it is daylight or darkness, and how long the days are.

Color: The Rainbow of Life

The opening paragraph of this chapter in Liberman's book is a powerful one that links light and life. He states that light brings to life the objects it touches and then these objects first appear as colors which become forms—our initial visual perceptions and discriminations are of color, then of form. Color has a power and language of its own. It causes us to feel excited, depressed, or peaceful. Used in advertising it can lead us to purchasing things. We speak of red hot, cool as a cucumber (green), white as a ghost, feeling blue, etc. Light is responsible for the emergence of all life, and all life literally is light.

Malillumination: Fact or Fancy

If light is the source of life as well as the major nutrient sustaining life, then poor or incomplete lighting must have an adverse affect on human life. Prior to the 1879 perfection of the incandescent bulb by Edison, most persons spent most of their time outdoors as most occupations and household chores like cutting wood, gardening, tending to animals, required an outdoor presence. Since that date increasing numbers of persons leaning on the illumination of the light bulb have spent ever-greater portions of each day indoors in a limited spectrum light environment.

The Enlightened Pioneers

Light's therapeutic applications and its affect on the function of all living things have been described by a number of persons since the days of Herodotus, the father of heliotherapy. There also have been a number of persons who have investigated the scientific properties of light.

A New Vision for Vision Specialists

The discovery of the successful treatment of bacterial infections with the first antibiotic, sulfanilamide, the "silver bullet" set the field of light therapy back into the field of witchcraft rather than of a non- intrusive miracle cure. Pharmaceutical companies pushed the new "wonder-drug" and it became the "magic pill" which would rid us of life threatening infections. Liberman laments, that we should have realized that it was our lifestyles, not bacteria, that caused disease. Our bodies are home to countless bacteria in balance within us. It is only when something occurs to create an imbalance that bacteria contribute to disease. (80)

Light, Color and Learning

It is a fact that for the sighted person, most learning occurs visually and that the eyes are the *major* entryway for light into the body. Since this is the case, what effect, if any, would modifying the general lighting and/or environmental color have in the school environment? In this chapter, Liberman cites the work of Dr. Harry Wohlfarth, Barbara M. Vitale, and Dr. Helen Irlen.

Light: Nature's Miracle Medicine

From ancient times people have recognized that cyclic or rhythmic patterns are an integral part of the functioning of all systems. In fact, these patterns are the basis for scientific predictions whose accuracy is contingent upon the assumption of orderly repetitiveness. Liberman asserts that this orderliness is "probably outside our universe" but eventually affects the tiniest atomic particle: from the universe to solar system—to earth—to the climate, seasons, inhabitants—to the tiniest atomic particle. (119)

179

Ultra Violet or Not Ultra Violet: That is the Question

Be cautious! Stay out of the sun. Protect yourself from exposure to *all* Ultraviolet light by using sun-blocking sunglasses, protective clothing, and sun block lotions at SPF 25 and 30.

These warnings are everywhere in the media and advertising. What are the real facts about sunlight?

It is generally agreed in scientific circles that ultraviolet light in *large* amounts is harmful, but according to Liberman, John Ott, and others, in *trace* amounts, as in natural light, ultraviolet light acts as a "life-supporting nutrient" (140).

Getting Well with the Rainbow Diet

Our entire blood supply circulates through our eyes about every two hours. Parts of the eye like the aqueous humor, lens, and vitreous humor, act as windows that allow light to directly stimulate the eyes and blood and to indirectly stimulate all other bodily functions…"every substance (vitamin, mineral, chemical, etcetera,) ingested by the body as food has a *maximum wavelength absorption characteristic*…for any ingested substance to be fully processed or used by the body, it needs to go through a series of chemical reactions that are catalyzed (ignited) by a specific portion of the electromagnetic spectrum" (157-158).

A New Paradigm for Health and Healing

It isn't germs and viruses that cause diseases, it is our lifestyles, the way we respond to stress, etc., that opens the door to imbalance and disease. Instead of focusing on killing microorganisms (like with antibiotics) we would be better off starving the offending microorganisms by changing our mental, emotional, and physical environments that *feed* these organisms. We need to concentrate our healing efforts on locating and dealing with the *causes* of our problems and not just on their effects. We need to deal with deep inner healing. (165-166)

Becoming Illuminated With Light

Thus, Liberman sets the scope for this chapter by reemphasizing that light is the basic tool needed to treat both the "within" (our emotional and mental states), and also the "without" (our functions and pathologies). (183)

He goes on to relate what he was taught in syntonics and how his experience with this light therapy caused him to develop new methods. He found that Spitler's original model of syntonics based on medical theories of the 1920's viewed the basis for dysfunctions and diseases primarily as the result of psychological imbalances rather than emotional ones. Liberman's book would demonstrate the opposite—emotional issues were primary and led to the imbalance that made the body vulnerable to dysfunction/disease.

Light: The Final Frontier

Liberman writes that, "Light is the superterrestrial, natural force under which all life on Earth originates and develops" (203). I would agree and add "Light is also *the* Supernatural Force (*above* and *before* nature). For Christians, Light centered in three Persons constituting one Divine Being is God.

Light therapy is a non-invasive technology unlike the commonest therapies of today, which involve powerful very invasive drugs with all kinds of undesirable side effects. At times it is a toss- up as to which is worse, the proposed cure or the disease! We are into the "light age." If Liberman is accurate in his predictions, "Scalpels will be replaced by lasers, chemotherapy by phototherapy, prescription drugs by prescription colors, acupuncture needles by needles of light, eye glasses by healthy eyes. Cancer will be a disease of the past"

(205).

A New Light on Cancer

In a "leading edge" paper written by engineer and inventor David Tumey and his associate, William Sheline, entitled "Royal Rife Revisited: Reconstruction of the Original Rife Ray Tube," the authors describe a fascinating piece of equipment and its related therapeutical uses.

Part Two:

The Conversation between Bernard Fleury and David Tumey in 2012–2013 reveals some new insights into engineer David Tumey's contracted services with regard to Rife Frequency Instruments and faster techniques for finding a desired mortal oscillatory rate.

Part Three:

The Amended Timeline of Royal R. Rife's Life reveals Rife's insights in his own words with regard to his life and accomplishments.

Part Four:

Royal Raymond Rife: Who? 1999-2014

There is renewed interest in Royal Rife's work in the Twenty First Century. First of all the American Medical Association, United States Research Hospitals and United States Pharmaceutical Companies do not have the same combined strangle-hold on doctors and hospitals working in Canada, England, France, Germany and Russia. Significant research has continued in these countries using Royal Rife's 1930's to1950's technology with updates from 2009 to 2014.

Endnotes

1   Jacob Liberman, *Light-Medicine of the Future* (Santa Fe, New Mexico: Bear and Company, 1991), p. xv. This and subsequent direct references from this work, are reprinted by permission of Inner Traditions International, Rochester, Vermont.

2   A. Szent-Gyorgyi, *Introduction in a Submolecular Biology* (New York: Academic Press, 1960). (cited in Liberman on pp. 8 & 9).

3   A. Szent-Gyorgyi, *Bioelectronics* (New York: Academic Press, 1968). (cited in Liberman on pp. 8 & 9).

4   K. Martinek and I.V. Berezin, "Artificial Light-Sensitive Enzymatic Systems as Chemical Amplifiers of Weak Light Signals", *Photochemistry and Photobiology* (29 March 1979), pp. 637-650. (cited in Liberman on p. 9).

5   Z. Kime, *Sunlight* (Penryn, California: World Health Publications, 1980). (cited by Liberman on p. 10).

6   Liberman, *op.cit.*, p. 14.

7   Peter A. Campbell and Edwin M. McMahon, *Bio-Spirituality* (Chicago Illinois: Loyola University Press, 1985), P.6. This and subsequent references for this work, are reprinted by permission of the publisher, Loyola University Press.

8   Campbell, *op.cit.*, p. 135.

9   R. Steiner, *Colour* (London: Rudolph Steiner Press, 1982). (cited by Liberman on p. 40).

10 Liberman, *op.cit.*, pp. 43-51.

11 J. N. Ott, "Color and Light: Their Effects on Plants, Animals

and People", *Journal of Biosocial Research* 7, part I (1985). (cited by Liberman on p. 58).

12 E. C. McBeath and T. F. Zuker, "The Role of Vitamin D in the Control of Dental Cavities in Children", *Journal of Nutrition* 15 (1938), p. 547. (cited by Liberman on p. 59).

13 B. R. East, "Mean Annual Hours of Sunshine and Incidence of Dental Cavities", *American Journal of Public Health* 29 (1939), p. 777. (cited by Liberman on p. 59).

14 L. Hays, "Which Came First, Low Cholesterol Egg or Happier Chicken", *The Wall Street Journal* 210, no, 113, (Dec. 8, 1987). (cited by Liberman on p. 59).

15 R. Altschul and I. H. Herman, "Ultraviolet Irradiation and Cholesterol Metabolism, Seventh Annual Meeting of the American Society for the Study of Arteriosclerosis", *Circulation* 8 (1853), p. 438. (cited by Liberman on p. 60).

16 Liberman, *op.cit.*, p. 61.

17 D. P. Ghadiali, *Spectro-Chrome Metry Encyclopedia* (Malaga, New Jersey: Spectro-Chrome Institute, 1933). (cited by Liberman on p. 72).

18 D. Dinshah, *Let There Be Light* (Malaga, New Jersey: Dinshah Health Society, 1985). (cited by Liberman on pp. 74-75).

19 H. R. Spitler, *The Syntonic Principle* (College of Syntonic Optometry, 1941). (cited by Liberman on p. 76).

20 Liberman, *op.cit.*, p. 81.

21 T. A. Brombach, *Visual Fields* (Transcript of Pictures, 1936). (cited by Liberman on p. 80).

22 T. .H. Eames, "Restrictions of the Visual Field as Handicaps to Learning", *Journal of Educational Research* 19 (Feb. 1936), pp. 460-63. (cited by Liberman on pp. 80-81).

23 T. H. Eames, "The Speed of Picture Recognition and the Speed of Word Recognition in Cases of Reading Difficulty", *American Journal of Ophthalmology* (21 Dec. 1958), pp. 1370-75. (cited by Liberman on pp. 80-81).

24 Liberman, *op.cit.*, p. 81.

25 Stephen Rae, "Bright Light, Big Therapy", *Modern Maturity* (Lakewood, California: American Association of Retired Persons, Vol. 37, #1 February – March 1994), p. 84.

26 Liberman, *op.cit.*, p. 122.

27 Rae. *op.cit.*, p. 38.

28 Liberman, *op.cit.*, p. 135.

29 R. M. Neer, et al., "Stimulation of Artificial Lighting of Calcium Absorption in Elderly Human Subjects", *Nature* 229 (1971), p. 255. (cited by Liberman on pp. 141-142).

30 Liberman, *op.cit.*, p. 140.

31 Zane R. Kime, M. D. Swannanoa Health Report, issues 2 and 3. (cited by Liberman on p. 155).

32 Campbell and McMahon. "What is Spiritual About Focusing"? (Coulterville, CA., Pamphlet Series, 1991), p. 1.

33 Liberman, *op.cit.*, p. 173.

34 David M. Tumey and William H. Sheline, "Royal Fife

Revisited: Reconstruction of the Original Rife Ray Tube" (Ohio: a paper written by the aforementioned authors describing their years of work researching and reconstructing a working replica of Royal Rife's Original Ray Tube apparatus, 1994), pp. 1-2.

Used with permission of David M. Tumey who sent the paper to me.

35 Liberman, *op.cit.*, p. 180.

36 David M. Tumey and William M. Sheline, "Royal Rife Revisited", pp. 1-2.

37 Robert P Stafford, "Electromagnetic Field Therapy", p. 1.

38 Liberman, *op.cit.,* pp. 111-112.

39 Stephen Rae, *op.cit.*, p. 84.

40 Liberman, *op.cit.*, pp. 115-116.

Bibliography

American Cancer Association,
http://www.cancer.org/cancer/pancreaticcancer/overvie
wguide/pancreatic-cancer-overview-survival-rates.

A New Light on Cancer: Sub Title in Part One: *The Medicine of Light,* in *The Mind-Body-Spirit Connection in the Medicine of Light,* Bernard J. Fleury, Called into Life by the Light Series, e-book Two, Amazon, December 2014.

Conversation on Royal Rife Ray Tube, David Tumey and Bernard J. Fleury, Called into Life by the Light Series, Part Two of e-book Two, Amazon, August 2014.

Dr. Royal R. Rife Speaks Again in the Year 2000, Edward Heft, Sr., Copyright holder, Kinneman Foundation, 2002.

Is Victory Over Pancreatic Cancer Possible With the Help of Tuned Non-Invasive Physiotherapy? A Case Study Says Yes.

Pierre Le Chapellier, Badri Matta, *Journal of Cancer Therapy,* 5, April 2014. An Abstract in Open Access Library.

Pancreatic Cancer Victory with PERL-M, The narrative of the full study. LeChapellier, B. Matta, *Journal of Cancer Therapy,* p. 464 (1), June 3, 2014.

Rife's World of Electromedicine, Barry Lynes, Bio Med Publishing Group, California, 2009. (Confirms and amplifies #3).

Royal Raymond Rife Discovers Cancer Cure, Jeff Rense, http://www.wanttoknow.info/cancercuresroyalrife, April 2003. (Confirms and amplifies #3).

The Annual Report of the Board of Regents of The Smithsonian Institution 1944, United States Government Printing Office, Washington, 1945.

The Cancer Cure That Worked, Barry Lynes, Bio Med Publishing Group, California, Thirteenth Printing May 2011. (Confirms and amplifies #3).

Video Picture Sources for e-book/audio book Trailer, Microscopes, Special Events, etcetera, are taken from:

—. http://www.facebook.com/RoyalRife

—. http://www.RifeDigital.com, Shannon Forbes, Nov. 11, 2014. (Permission granted)

—. http://www.resonantlight.com (with permission of owner, Edna Anne Tunney), Nov. 7, 2014.

Epilogue

The Mind-Body-Spirit Connection in The Medicine of Light

This e-book/audio book presented comprehensive examples of how the Mind-Body-Spirit Connection in the Medicine of Light affects current medical practice and technology that promotes the well being of every person who is fortunate enough to have experienced the use of at least some of the light based therapies and devices in the diagnosis and treatment for one or more of his/her ailments.

Parts Two, Three, and Four also reveal the ongoing conflict between the United States medical establishment and some important parts of Royal R. Rife's technology based on rigidly clinging to a view of the living body as basically chemical in opposition to modern physics' view that the living body is basically electrical (forms of light). Unfortunately, after years of reading and experience documented in Part Four, I have to add greed, loss of power, unwillingness to change are also basic reasons for the continuing conflict.

The American Medical Association (AMA) and the Food and Drug Administration (FDA) require a **series** of clinical trials that have approved results and are therefore considered to be successful. Nearly all clinical trials require some sort of pharmaceutical (drug) inclusion. (After all, who funds most of the "clinical" trials!) Then you can play around with "alternative medicine" therapies that the American Medical Association, Food and Drug Administration, and Pharmaceutical Companies will accept as complementary and secondary to "standard practice".

Why is Royal Raymond Rife's name, technology, therapies, etcetera., unknown to the overwhelming majority of United States Medical Doctors?

Royal Rife's well documented discoveries threatened a very comfortable status quo world for the bureaucratic, civil servants, and regulators who lived there.

Medical school textbooks and courses were wiped clean of any reference to him.

Some Medical Doctors admitted they were pawns of the drug industry. Two of my Physician Assistants and three of my Medical Doctors admit the overwhelming influence of Pharmaceutical Companies on Medical Societies.

Honest testing that utilized Rife's Universal Microscope was never done by those designated by the National Health Organizations in trying to replicate his claims. Continued denial of pleomorphism in the United States, even though it had been proven over and over by Rife and the well known and eminent doctors who worked with him during his lifetime. Some of these doctors continued using his technology after his death in 1971 in the United States, Germany and France.

I also discovered in discussion with my doctors during hospital stays and office visits that they had very little formal education in Physics, often no more than common core undergraduate courses. All of these doctors have excellent reputations in their respective medical specialties or as General Practitioners.

Good news, my readers, there is new light peeping over the horizon. The internet is coming alive. There is a founded hope that change will occur if enough of the public demands it. When I was doing a final niche research on Amazon entering "Royal R. Rife" on November 14, 2014, I found fifty one entries. E-book Two, The Mind-Body-Spirit Connection in The Medicine of Light in the Called into Life Series of e-books and audio/books will be the newest entry for January 2015 for Royal Rife and for the title of e-book Two.

I invite you to join me as we move on now to e-book Three in our Called into Life by the Light Series. What does *The Search for the Light in Evolution* reveal about my place as a human person in the development of the earth?

Made in the USA
Monee, IL
23 February 2020